VITAMINS, MINERALS AND DIETARY SUPPLEMENTS

A definitive guide to healthy eating

Hasnain Walji

 *eadway* · Hodder & Stoughton

Note: Information given in this book is not intended to be taken as a replacement for medical advice. Any person with a condition requiring medical attention should consult a medical professional.

Cataloguing in Publication Data is available from the British Library

Walji, Hasnain
  Vitamins, Minerals and Dietary Supplements: Definitive Guide to
  Healthy Eating. – (Definitive Guides)
  I. Title II. Series
  613.28

ISBN 0 340 61905 8

First published 1995
Impression number 10 9 8 7 6 5 4 3 2
Year   1998   1997   1996

Printed in Great Britain for Hodder & Stoughton Educational, a division of Hodder Headline Plc, 338 Euston Road, London NW1 3BH by Cox & Wyman Ltd, Reading.

$\mathcal{C}$ONTENTS

INDEX OF CONDITIONS

$\mathcal{P}$REFACE

If you are fit and healthy and *know* that you are getting all the nutrients you need from a 'well balanced diet' then you do not need this book. Pass it to someone you know who looks run down and seems to be constantly tired or who appears to be lacking vitality and enthusiasm. Maybe you know someone who suffers from insomnia, low sex drive, premenstrual syndrome, or one of the many other diseases of the twentieth century who could benefit from this book. However, if any of the above *do* apply to you, then read on.

This *Definitive Guide to Vitamins, Minerals and Dietary Supplements* has been written specifically to be a handy reference to demystify the subject of healthy eating. The Introduction explains why we need vitamins and minerals and how to determine correct amounts for optimum health. It discusses the link between today's modern diseases and nutrition and helps you determine if vitamin and mineral supplements are necessary for you. The indexes that follow on from the Introduction describe the vitamins, minerals and other dietary supplements, explain what they do, what the deficiency symptoms are, and, most important of all, the best sources from which they can be obtained. Finally, the index of common ailments, which covers the role of nutrition in controlling many deficiency diseases as well other twentieth century ailments, such as heart disease and stress, will give you all the information you will need about the role of diet in combatting illness.

Correct nutrition can do much to enhance life and maintain health. This easy-to-read guide will enable you to make an intelligent choice of health-promoting foods or supplements, whether you are in the supermarket or confronted by a plethora of pills in a health food store. More importantly, it will help you to take positive action on attaining health and well-being rather than just curing a disease. Remember, health is not just absence of disease but a positive sense of well-being.

Hasnain Walji
Milton Keynes, September 1994

6

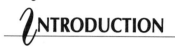

INTRODUCTION

*W*HY DO WE NEED VITAMINS AND MINERALS?

The human body needs a well-balanced diet that provides all the nutrients in the right proportions. All foods contain varying amounts of nutrients. Proteins, carbohydrates and fats, called macronutrients, are generously provided in abundance by the modern Western diet and form the bulk of the food that we eat. Vitamins and minerals, known as micronutrients, are present in very small quantities in all natural vegetable and animal food. Vitamins and minerals feature as vital ingredients in a healthy diet and the body cannot function optimally if they are missing. Nutritionists believe that in the West we are deficient in some micronutrients and that this is affecting our health.

FUNCTION OF VITAMINS AND MINERALS

Very simply, vitamins and minerals do not contain calories, nor do they provide energy. It is the macronutrients that do this. However, this energy cannot be properly released without vitamins and minerals. In other words vitamins and minerals, being part of enzymes, are organic catalysts which allow the release of energy, thus stimulating the metabolic process and accelerating biological functions. Indeed, human life without enzymes and vitamins would be impossible as they are responsible for converting our food into energy. Vitamins are also involved in promoting growth and maintaining the immune function. They enable reproduction to take place and promote longevity.

In addition, minerals are also important for healthy bones and teeth. Like vitamins, minerals cannot be manufactured by the body and must also come from the diet.

HOW MUCH?

While we all need the same vitamins and minerals for good health and well-being, individual requirements vary with age, sex, lifestyle and occupation. It is because of this that there can be no standard formula to determine individual requirements. There are tables that give average nutrient requirements but these are largely inadequate because of the manner in which they have been calculated. Although the tables are revised from time to time they do not contain all known nutrients and are therefore incomplete. These tables give Recommended Daily Allowances (RDA).

RDA levels are calculated by observing statistically the average food intake of healthy individuals and calculating the vitamin/mineral content. For good measure, a safety margin is added to compile the tables. These tables cannot take into account specific and individual needs caused by the different stages in one's life, or indeed specific conditions such as stress, allergies or environmental pollution. Standards in the form of Recommended Intakes for Nutrients (DHSS 1969) and Recommended Daily Allowances (DHSS 1979) have existed in the UK for over thirty years. However, many people have not understood how they have been derived, how they are intended to be used and the degree of accuracy that ought to be attributed to them. In particular, the RDAs have been (incorrectly) used to assess the inadequacy of an individual's diet.

Therefore, in order to overcome the 'abuses' of the figures and to update them in the light of recent information and research, the Department of Health asked the Committee on Medical Aspects of Food Policy (COMA) to set up a panel of experts to look at the matter. As a result, a new set of updated figures, collectively known as Dietary Reference Values, has been established. So instead of simple RDA figures we now have four different sets of figures for each nutrient. These are:

- Estimated Average Requirement;
- Recommended Nutrient Intake;
- Lowest Nutrient Intake;
- Safe Intake.

The publication of these new dietary guidelines reflects the fact that at long last the health authorities have accepted that some people need more of one nutrient than others.

CORRECT AMOUNTS FOR OPTIMAL HEALTH

There is no question that we all need nutrients in the correct amounts for optimal health. What is difficult is to determine what these amounts are. For example, a pregnant woman has higher dietary needs of certain nutrients, while adolescents require greater quantities of some nutrients to ensure growth and development. The elderly need extra nutrients to counteract the effects of ageing, and a busy executive under stress needs more of certain nutrients to offset the damaging effects that stress has on the whole body.

The Dietary and Nutritional Survey of British Adults (HMSO, 1990) illustrates that although the average intake of vitamins and minerals in the UK population is usually adequate, there are significant numbers of subgroups of the population that have extremely marginal intakes. According to this report 2.5 per cent of British women between the ages of 25 and 34 are only getting 11.8mg of vitamin C or less per day. The recommended figure for this group is 40mg.

Similar statistics exist for many other nutrients. In many cases it is women rather than men who fall short of vitamins and minerals; but there are instances where 2.5 per cent of the population (both men and women) fall below the Recommended Daily Allowance. This may not appear significant, but what it means in real terms is that 1.4 million British people are deficient in one or several nutrients.

TODAY'S MODERN DISEASES AND NUTRITION

There is little dispute that diet is linked to the increase in the incidence of major degenerative diseases such as heart disease, osteoporosis, cancer and many others. For example, vitamin C has been linked to warding off the common cold, the vitamin B-complex with a healthy nervous system, and garlic with lowering blood cholesterol. Vitamins and minerals do not just offer day-to-day benefits. There is growing evidence to suggest that some of these micronutrients, called antioxidants, can help prevent the long-term illnesses such as cancer. Vitamins C, E, and beta carotene, and minerals zinc and selenium, are now considered to be the main players in this regard, with fruits and vegetables being the best source of these. For example, even marginal deficiencies of vitamins A, C, E, and B6 have been shown to increase susceptibility to a number of viral and bacterial infections. Research indicates that these vitamins help maintain our immune systems, as deficiency can impair the body's ability to resist disease. Antioxidants prevent oxygen from combining with other substances and thus damaging cells.

Many of the B vitamins play a vital role in releasing energy from the cells, and stress depletes them much more quickly from the body. The first part of the body to be affected by a mild vitamin B deficiency is the nervous system, resulting in anxiety, irritability and depression.

Minerals act as cofactors and catalysts inside the human cells and have far-reaching effects on our health, too. Until recently only calcium, phosphorus, iron and iodine were recognised as being essential minerals for human health. As research continues, zinc, chromium, magnesium, potassium, manganese and selenium have all been been shown to be necessary for human health. New findings bring to light many ailments caused by mineral deficiencies. Take PMS as an example. Many women find that just by altering their diet so that it contains more magnesium and zinc, their symptoms can be decreased. Among others, positive results have been achieved with selenium and rheumatoid arthritis, with zinc and skin problems, and with calcium and osteoporosis.

As research continues, the importance of maintaining optimum levels of nutrient intake becomes increasingly evident.

WHERE TO FIND THE NUTRIENTS

The most important question of all, however, is whether we are getting all the nutrients we need from our food. It is commonly believed that we can get all the vitamins and minerals we need if we eat a well-balanced diet. But what is a well-balanced diet, and is it easy and practical to follow? How many times do we skip breakfast as we rush to work? How often do we grab a pizza or hamburger as we dash back to the office after shopping or paying the gas bill during our lunch hour? As we return in the evening, a take-away is tempting because we are too tired to cook.

It is important to realise that vitamins cannot, by definition, be manufactured by the body and must therefore come from the diet. A vitamin is a delicate, unstable entity that can easily be destroyed during its transportation from the farm to the factory to the supermarket. The little that is left is often lost in its journey from the freezer to the microwave to the table.

Our supermarkets may have cheap, plentiful food, but the economics of the food industry have also adversely affected the quality of the food we eat. Modern farming techniques mean that not only is our food grown in chemicals but is also covered in them. After harvesting, produce is treated to give it an extended life to survive the transport, storage and shelf times required by today's food manufacturers. We then store the food at home and often use cooking methods that destroy any vitamin or mineral content which may have been remaining. It is ironic that the typical Western diet is lacking in sufficient quantities of essential nutrients and that we may be *overfed* but still remain *undernourished*.

ARE VITAMIN AND MINERAL SUPPLEMENTS NECESSARY?

How do we ensure that we are not undernourished despite being overfed? In an ideal world our food would supply us with the nutrients we require. While we should strive for the ideal, we also need to be realistic. While we need to improve our eating habits, food alone cannot be sufficient for a majority of us. It is not sufficient because, however nutrient-packed the original product, refining, storing, processing, freezing, and even exposure to the air, all take their toll in the depletion of essential nutrients. Furthermore, each individual has his or her own nutritional requirements, some of which may exceed the amount that could possibly be ingested from even the healthiest of diets. Then there are the ravages of stress, illness, pollution and the extra demands of young children, pregnant women and breast-feeding mothers. A wholesome diet plus supplements is an approach that will ensure that we get the correct amount of nutrients required for optimum health.

Dr Willard A Krehl, of Jefferson Medical College, and Editor in Chief of the American *Journal of Clinical Nutrition,* says

'My own bias on the value of nutrient supplementation has developed over the years through my experience in clinical practice. I continually see that in spite of the fact that our clients are generally in the executive category and can therefore purchase an excellent diet, most of them do not eat properly. For whatever reasons, most of them skip breakfast or eat the wrong things for breakfast; they have a fast food lunch high in fat and often low in micronutrients; they consume a good deal of sugar, sweets and alcoholic beverages. In short, my search for the individuals who consistently eat a well-balanced, varied and nutritionally adequate diet has merely impressed me with the fact that millions of people do not ..... I strongly favour multi vitamin supplementation and recommend it to my patients because I believe it is a simple, economical, and highly practical way to ensure they receive 100 per cent of the RDA for essential micronutrients, and because I believe these intakes are important to health and well-being.'

He concludes that

'... the high incidence of below RDA micronutrient intakes, resulting from multiple factors including poor food choices, decreased caloric intakes and personal/environmental/lifestyle factors, presents a situation where multi vitamin supplementation is both a rational and beneficial choice. Supplementation provides a practical and economic means of ensuring adequate nutrient intakes and is of particular importance to risk groups such as dieters, the elderly, heavy drinkers, chronic drug users and others whose diets are insufficient or whose ability to utilise food is impaired. Therefore there is really no reason to tolerate nutrient deficiencies when such a simple and sensible alternative as

supplementation exists. It must, however, be emphasised that
supplements cannot replace a wholesome diet, but can augment a
bad one.'

WHICH SUPPLEMENTS?

Due care must be taken in choosing supplements. The general
multi vitamin mineral supplements are usually one-a-day pills
that contain carefully graded amounts of nutrients and may
serve as an 'insurance policy'. The single vitamin and mineral
supplements are normally used for specific conditions. These
must only be taken in consultation with a dietary therapist or a
professional nutritional counsellor. Temptation to take higher
than stated doses should be resisted as it is possible, in extreme
cases, to overdose on vitamins and minerals. Your health
food store or pharmacy will have a great many pills, potions and
powders on the shelves. So which one do you choose? To
confuse you even further, the labels do not just say 'Vitamin C'
or 'Iron' but have adjectives like 'chelated', 'timed-release',
'divided dose' and 'high potency'. What does it all mean?

A multi vitamin–mineral supplement

A well-balanced multi vitamin–mineral preparation may be all
that you need. In conjunction with expert advice, it can be
taken with single nutrients added for those with specific needs.

- Choose a multi vitamin–mineral preparation.
- Unless individual nutrients have been prescribed by a
  nutritionist or a doctor, avoid taking numerous individual
  supplements.

A multi vitamin–mineral should contain at least the following
nutrients: vitamin A, beta carotene, B-complex, vitamins C, D,
E, and the minerals phosphorous, calcium, magnesium,
potassium, iron, zinc, manganese, copper, iodine, molybdenum,
chromium, selenium, vanadium.
　　The better multi vitamin–mineral preparations also contain
additional nutrients, such as choline, inositol, methionine,

PABA, bioflavonoids, lysine, lecithin, rutin, betaine, hesperdine and cysteine.

High potency vitamins

Do not be misled into thinking that 'more is better'. Most vitamins and minerals work in the body in conjunction with enzymes. In most cases consuming more than the required amount will not increase the metabolic activity. Instead the body will either store the excess nutrient if it is fat soluble (vitamin A or D), or it will be flushed out if it is water soluble (vitamin C). Megadoses of the fat-soluble vitamins A and D over long periods of time can produce toxic effects and can also interfere with the absorption and use of other nutrients.

Timed-release supplements

Timed-release, continuous action and sustained release are synonymous terms denoting a process whereby the ingredients of a tablet are trickled out of a binding matrix. In contrast to a conventional tablet, which releases all of the ingredients within a short period of time, timed-release tablets release small quantities over a prolonged period. This process is particularly useful in the case of water-soluble vitamins.

Chelated minerals

A chelated mineral is one that is chemically bound to another substance. This can involve a number of substances but in nature it is usually a protein or group of amino acids. Although research is as yet inconclusive, it is generally accepted that amino acid chelates are absorbed in far greater amounts than any other mineral form. Their absorption is at least three, and in some cases up to ten, times the amount of non-chelated forms.

Natural or organic

The words 'natural' or 'organic' have little to offer except increased cost in case of supplements. The process of extracting nutrients from foods can hardly be termed natural and in many cases chemical solvents are used to extract and purify them.

Bioavailability

This term refers to the amount of an ingested nutrient that is absorbed and utilised by the body. Just swallowing a multi vitamin supplement does not mean that a person will benefit from the full quantity of the nutrients in the pill. Unless the nutrients are consumed in optimal ratios to other nutrients it will not have the maximum absorption from the digestive tract into the blood stream. Additionally, the nutrient must be ingested in a form that the body can convert for use in the metabolic process. Poorly made supplements may pass through the body without even dissolving.

Bioavailability of a supplement is affected by other dietary components. For example, a high intake of fibre will inhibit calcium absorption. Supplementing diets with large amounts of iron or zinc may inhibit the absorption of some trace minerals. This is because the minerals compete with each other for absorption. When one is provided in abundance, a secondary deficiency of another mineral may result.

OVERDOSING AND TOXICITY

Anything can be harmful if taken in excess. Even water can kill if too much is drunk. Vitamins and minerals are among the safest substances that anyone can take and the amounts for them to be toxic have to be enormous.

The general definition of a megadose is a dose of the nutrient which is at least ten times the average RDA. Megavitamins are necessary when the body is unable to absorb adequate quantities of vitamins in the stomach, or in certain cases where vitamins do not function properly in the body.

*N*UTRIENT DENSITY

The nutrient content of different foods as compared to their caloric content is the basis of what dietitians call 'nutrient density'. Some foods are naturally healthy to consume, with a high nutrient value in relation to their caloric (energy) content. A fundamental rule of diet planning to promote health is to choose foods with a high nutrient density. Problems arise when needed nutrients are missing from a diet, as well as when too many calories are consumed for daily energy needs. Whole grains and beans provide enough B vitamins to help process the energy they contain, and, therefore, are of proper nutrient density. A white flour, high-fat food may contain more calories than its nutrient value can handle and this robs health.

- All food fats have 9 calories per gram and carbohydrates and proteins both contain 4 calories per gram, or roughly half of the calories by weight. Fats provide the fat-soluble vitamins A, D, E and K. Some fat is necessary for these vitamins' absorption. However, most people eat far too much fat.
- Sweets and fats appear in the diet because they are pleasurable to eat. Salad dressing decreases the nutrient density of the salad and soured cream decreases the nutrient density of a baked potato. You will need to identify and avoid these and a few other traps in making food selection. Learn the basics of food selection and apply them every minute of a meal.

The following tips should help:

- target fats, sweets, and salt as your health enemies. Enjoy them in moderation only, if at all. Imagine a clogged artery in 20 years to help avoid low-nutrient-density foods today;
- substitute skinless chicken and white fish for red meat;
- start a vegetarian cookbook collection or visit the local library for recipes;
- when eating out, select 'healthy' restaurants if possible. Most restaurant staff are very understanding when asked to poach fish, and to provide salad dressings separately. Many people are already eating out healthily. Some fast food restaurants have introduced 'healthier' selections, but always watch out for fat, sugar and salt;
- as a general rule, shop on the outside of the supermarket aisles, avoiding the processed foods which are heavily

merchandised on the interior of the store. Fresh produce, lean meats and fish are generally found lining the store;

- check Yellow Pages, actively shop and ask friends about well-stocked stores for fresh produce and natural foods. Become aware of which vegetables are coming into season for long-term diet planning. Trade recipes with friends and try them out on each other. Cooking with a purpose makes a hobby out of a daily chore. Good cooking skills will give you control over eating healthily. Make a commitment to become a better cook, practise actively, don't place unrealistic expectations on yourself, and acknowledge your accomplishments, however small.

$\mathcal{C}$XERCISE AND SPORTS

The human body was designed to be exercised. The heart is a muscular pump, which needs the stimulation of increased workloads to stay healthy over long periods of time. Research is continually finding new relationships between the role of exercise and optimal health. How much exercise is enough? This question is hotly debated, and some findings suggest that regular, mild exercise is best and anything above this level may not help promote health.

Many of us ignore exercise for a number of reasons, but top researchers into ageing quote the saying, 'The body doesn't wear out .... it rusts out.' Inactivity will definitely shorten an individual's maximum genetic lifespan, and even mild, regular exercise will add to a positive mental outlook and sense of well-being. Exercise has been proven to lower blood triglycerides and raise the HDL (good) cholesterol ratio, both of which reduce the risk of heart disease. Many degenerative diseases are related to obesity and exercise keeps off extra pounds.

Exercise physiologists know that as we age, we gradually lose our ability to perform work. For the average person, part of this decline is due to the biochemical changes of ageing and part is due to under use. The body will adapt to the stress of exercise by increasing its ability to perform work output, an effect that is vital to employ during the younger years to ensure a healthy old age. Proper nutrition will delay or minimise the biochemical changes of ageing that create degenerative diseases and will make exercise and recovery much more enjoyable.

Depending on the age a person begins a regular exercise programme, they will want to engage in activities that make their heart beat in a 'target range' above their resting pulse rate. If the exercise is too moderate or too brief, the heart isn't benefiting from the activity and if the pulse is forced above the high range, overstressing can occur. A physical examination by a health professional is recommended for determining health status and ideal pulse range.

The goal of an exercise programme is to achieve the state of maximum conditioning; this will vary with age and genetic potential. When a person becomes short of breath during exercise, the body is trying to produce more energy than the oxygen supply will allow. When physical output is continued past this point, muscles go into a condition of oxygen debt and change from anaerobic (without oxygen) metabolism. The energy to power the muscles is now coming from a less efficient pathway that produces lactic acid in the muscles and this creates the familiar 'burning' sensation. Because of this effect, exercise intensity is best increased slowly, allowing the body time to adapt to the new and necessary stresses it creates.

Warning
If you are planning on starting an exercise programme, you should consult with a health care professional.

LIGHT EXERCISE

Nutritional needs will not change for a person engaging in regular, light exercise. Bicycling, walking etc., do not put great demands on the healthy body and will contribute benefits through relaxation and blood oxygenation. If a person engages in work that requires continuous light exercise, he or she will want to pay attention to fluid and mineral electrolyte intake, especially in hot and/or humid weather. Fruits and vegetables,

both rich in potassium, should be emphasised in the diet.
Hunger should match caloric output to achieve energy balance.
As always, nutritious wholegrain carbohydrates, such as breads,
pastas, and grain dishes, should supply calories for exercise
because fat and protein calories should stay constant.
Carbohydrates are more readily burned and are stored in the
muscle as glycogen, which eases recovery.

MEDIUM EXERCISE

The conversion of food (fuel) into energy is continually driving
our hearts and expanding our lungs, even during sleep.
Engaging in regular, medium intensity exercise places demands
on the body's ability to deliver oxygen and fuel (carbohydrate
and fats) to the active muscle groups. The well-exercised body
rewards itself by being calm, less susceptible to stress and
feeling positive. Having a leaner, healthier, more attractive body
will yield long-term benefits in self-image as well.

Physically active occupations, such as gardening,
construction, etc., require thoughtful food choices to ensure
adequate nutrient density in proportion to calorie content.
Among many, the B vitamins are especially important in energy
production serving as the 'spark' that releases the stored energy
in food fuels. A history of consuming calorie dense/nutrient
poor foods, such as concentrated sweets, refined grains and
alcohol, will create problems because the body will exhaust B
vitamin reserves in energy production without any nutritional
payback.

HEAVY EXERCISE

As the human body adapts to the vigours of exercise, it
becomes better able to perform at higher levels of intensity.
Heavy exercise can stress the body's ability to recover from the
accumulated damage to tissues and can actually decrease
athletic performance in trained athletes. At this level of training,
rest intervals and cross-training become very important and
professional coaching helps by giving objective feedback.

More than average protein is required to support the muscle

mass increase for body building. Multiple nutritional supplementation is recommended to support the great metabolic demands placed on the body by growing new muscle tissue. As runners and cyclists achieve a lean physique, their bodies contain less fat storage for energy production. Training becomes dependent on supplying the muscles with enough carbohydrates to replace glycogen levels that are rapidly used during this time. Nutrient-dense carbohydrate foods assume great importance for endurance athletes, both for successful training and winning competition. Competition at the highest level places a great stress on the body and skilled coaching is necessary to avoid overtraining.

Some world-class athletes employ, among others, supplements like ginseng to reduce the immune suppression caused by pushing the body to its physical limits and beyond. Other supplements can assist the body in delivering oxygen and fuel (glucose or fatty acids) to the muscle at a maximal rate. As a rule, performance-enhancing supplementation should be used sparingly during training and just before competition, to ensure their application is consistent with biochemical goals.

$\mathcal{W}$EIGHT LOSS AND DIETING

Diet and exercise are partners in the pursuit of a leaner, healthier body. Most people, in theory, have complete control over their eating behaviour and exercise habits, but the success of the commercial weight-loss industry reveals a need for guidance and educational input. Through self-education and the wilful application of this knowledge, anyone can achieve results in reaching their weight-loss goals.

Some diet strategies advocate the avoidance of, or emphasis on one type of food. Some require buying expensive prepared foods. Neither of these strategies is correct because, at best, it allows a short-term correction of a long-term problem. Weight lost is very easily regained in so called 'yo-yo' diets because all behavioural and biochemical factors are not considered.

- **Fact 1** The body has a given number of fat storage (adipose) cells that increase or decrease in size to accommodate changing levels of fat storage.
- **Fact 2** Dietary fats are very easily stored in the adipose cells and for this reason a low-fat diet must be employed to reduce existing body fat stores.
- **Fact 3** For successful weight loss, dietary fats should be reduced gradually to the minimum tolerable level. This will be around 20 per cent of calories for most people. Any lower and meals will not be satisfying, due to the rapid release from the stomach to the intestine and the rapid onset of hunger. A gradual, conscious decrease will be necessary to avoid discomfort and ensure a successful long-term change in eating habits.
- **Fact 4** Because dietary fats are so satisfying, they occur everywhere in prepared foods. A diet of carefully prepared grains, fruits and vegetables is ideal. Fats from coldwater fish and olive oil are actually good for the body and should ideally comprise the majority of fat calories. Fats from animal sources (i.e. flesh and dairy products) are less healthy and should be taken at a minimum. Do this by eating vegetable protein, skinless chicken and fish. Remember, dietary fat is your weight-loss enemy today and your heart disease enemy long term. Work constantly to keep fat calories at a minimum.

    Adopt fat reduction strategies such as avoiding restaurants without healthy selections on the menu and ordering sauces and salad dressing separately. By studying food labels in the supermarket, one can rapidly become aware of the fat content of foods. All food labels must list ingredients in order of amount, so healthier foods will show fat as one of the last few ingredients. Butter, margarine, shortening, lard, and oils are all fat sources found in processed foods and recipes. Start collecting recipes and cookbooks focused on low-fat foods.
- **Fact 5** All foods will become fat storage if they are consumed in excess of energy needs. Protein and fat needs are most often fixed in humans, and complex carbohydrates should contribute energy (calories) as needed. To reduce

body fat stores, more energy needs to be used in daily activities and exercise than is consumed from foods. The nutrient content of foods must be high, especially if fewer calories are consumed. Sweet foods (simple carbohydrates) should be avoided because of the low nutrient density and high fat content often found in them.

- **Fact 6** Very-low-calorie diets without exercise contribute to the burning of muscle mass as well as body fat. This condition is very unhealthy for the body and rebound hunger results in the regaining of body fat. The body regains fat more easily and over time changes the body composition to a higher percentage of fat. The correct approach is gradually to increase the exercise output while, at the same time, gradually decreasing the calorie intake. Fast change does not work in the long term.
- **Fact 7** A well-exercised body will be biochemically 'trained' to utilise fats more efficiently from the diet and from storage as energy sources. The tendency to store fats is reduced with increasing levels of athletic training. If the exercise intensity is high enough, the body will burn energy for hours after the exercise stops. This effect increases the Basal Metabolic Rate (BMR) which is the energy one burns at rest. Without the exercise-induced increase in BMR, dieting for body-fat loss becomes an exercise in futility.

*R*ECOMMENDED NUTRIENT INTAKES

Standards in the form of Recommended Intakes for Nutrients and Recommended Daily Amounts of food energy and nutrients have existed in the UK for over thirty years.

In order to update them in the light of more recent information, the Department of Health's Chief Medical Officer asked the Committee on Medical Aspects of Food Policy (COMA) to set up a panel of experts to consider the matter. The panel revised the standards and came up with the following new standards.

Estimated Average Requirement (EAR)

The panel's estimate of the average requirement or need for food energy or a nutrient. Clearly, many people will need more than the average and many people will need less.

Reference Nutrient Intake (RNI)

An amount of a nutrient that is enough for almost every individual, even someone who has high needs for the nutrient. This level of intake is, therefore, considerably higher than most people need. If individuals are consuming the RNI of a nutrient they are most unlikely to be deficient in that nutrient. **RNIs are equivalent in definition to the old RDAs.**

Lower Reference Nutrient Intake (LRNI)

The amount of a nutrient that is enough for only the small number of people with low needs. Most people will need more than the LRNI if they are to eat enough. If individuals are habitually eating less than the LRNI they will almost certainly be deficient.

Safe Intake

A term normally used to indicate the intake of a nutrient for which there is not enough information to estimate requirements. A safe intake is one that is judged to be adequate for almost everyone's needs, but not so large as to cause undesirable effects.

*M*AJOR RECOMMENDATIONS ON DIET

ENERGY

The energy needs of people in the UK, as estimated by the COMA panel, are shown on the next page:

ESTIMATED AVERAGE REQUIREMENTS FOR ENERGY (KCAL*/DAY)		
Age	Males	Females
0–3 months	545	515
4–6 months	690	645
7–9 months	825	765
10–12 months	920	865
1–3 years	1230	1165
4–6 years	1715	1545
7–10 years	1970	1740
11–14 years	2220	1845
15–18 years	2755	2110
19–50 years	2550	1940
51–59 years	2500	1900
60–64 years	2380	1900
65–74 years	2330	1900
75+ years	2110	1810

The above figures for energy were based on present low activity levels. There was broad agreement that an increase in energy expenditure was necessary for the population as a whole, which, if achieved, would mean an increase in the figures given above.

* See Glossary on page 139

CARBOHYDRATES

The recommendations of the committee were that about 37 per cent of the energy content of the diet should come from starches, intrinsic sugars and lactose (milk sugar). Anybody obtaining less than this percentage of their energy from these carbohydrate sources was probably relying too heavily on fat and protein as an energy source.

It was felt by the panel that no more than 10 per cent of the energy content of the diet should be derived from extrinsic sugars (e.g. sweets and confectionery), as above that level there were attendant risks of dental decay, etc.

FIBRE

The panel proposed that the average intake of fibre (measured as non-starch polysaccharides) should be 18g per day in adults, with an expected range of individual intakes from 12–24g, depending on body size.

A review of fibre intakes showed that greater than 32g per day of non-starch polysaccharides was not associated with any ill-effects. However, the possibility that the phytate content of fibre may bind minerals and make them unavailable to the body should not be overlooked.

PROTEIN

The 1991 COMA figures for protein, based on recommendations from the World Health Organisation, are quite a bit lower than previous recommendations. This is because in the past figures had been based on the fact that people in the UK obtained at least 10 per cent of their energy as protein rather than on how much the body actually needed. It was felt that the maximum protein intake for a normal person should not exceed twice the RNI. The exception may be very active people or those engaged in strength sports.

FAT

The panel decided that the specific types of fat eaten were more important than the total fat consumed. Hence it is conceivable that someone with a high total fat intake could be at a lower health risk than someone with a lower total fat intake – purely because of a difference in the types of fat eaten.

The COMA recommendations on fat are shown on the chart on the next page:

Age	(g/day)	Age	(g/day)
0-3 months	12.5	15-18 years (males)	55.2
4-6 months	12.7	15-18 years (females)	45.4
7-9 months	13.7	19-49 years (males)	55.5
10-12 months	14.9	19-49 years (females)	45.0
1-3 years	14.5	50+ years (males)	53.3
4-6 years	19.7	50+ years (females)	46.5
7-10 years	28.3	Pregnancy	51.0
11-14 years (males)	42.1	Lactation (0-6months)	56.0
11-14 years (females)	41.2	(6+ months)	53.0

- The total fat content of the diet should on average provide 33 per cent of the total energy intake.
- No more than 10 per cent of the total energy intake should come from saturated fatty acids.
- Approximately 6 per cent of the total energy intake should come from polyunsaturated fatty acids.
- Approximately 12 per cent of the total energy intake should come from monounsaturated fatty acids.
- Trans-fatty acids (found in heat processed oils) should provide no more than 2 per cent of the total energy intake.

$\mathcal{V}$ITAMINS AND MINERALS

The 1991 COMA report also details recommendations for daily intakes of many vitamins and minerals. These are dealt with separately in the appropriate parts of this book.

*I*NDEX OF VITAMINS

$\mathcal{V}$ITAMIN A

Did you know?

- Vitamin A occurs in two forms – preformed vitamin A, known as retinol, and provitamin A, known as beta carotene.
- Vitamin A is known as the vision vitamin, for its role in aiding eyesight.
- Vitamin A is fat soluble – it is stored in the liver and need not be replenished every day.

Benefits

- Vitamin A helps maintain healthy skin, teeth and bones and mucous membranes in the nose, throat and lungs.
- It is necessary in the formation of an eye pigment involved in night vision, and is essential for vision in dim light.
- Vitamin A is needed for proper development of the foetus in the womb.

Deficiency symptoms

- Severe deficiency leads to various physical changes in the eye and will eventually lead to blindness.
- Marginal deficiency will lead to increased susceptibility to respiratory tract infections and skin problems.

Measurement

- IU (international units) or RE (retinol equivalents)

Requirements (RNI)

THE RNI VALUES (COMA 1991) FOR VITAMIN A					
Age	(mcg/day)	(iu/day)	Age	(mcg/day)	(iu/day)
0–12 months	350	1167	11–14 years (male)	600	2000
1–6 years	400	1333	15+ years (male)	700	2333
7–10 years	500	1667	Pregnancy	700	2333
11+ years (female)	600	2000	Lactation	950	3167

Best food sources

- Liver, carrots, milk, margarine and butter.

Food	Retinol (mcg/100g)	(iu/100g)	Food	Retinol (mcg/100g)	(iu/100g)
Halibut liver oil	900000	3000000	Eggs	190	633
Lamb's liver	19900	66333	Pig's kidney	160	533
Cod liver oil	18000	60000	Milk	56	187
Butter	985	3283	Mackerel	45	150
Margarine	800	2667	Beef	10	33
Cheese, Cheddar	363	1210	Sardines, canned	7	23

Who may need to supplement

- Vegetarians.
- Diabetics (who cannot efficiently convert beta carotene into vitamin A).
- Those with fat malabsorption syndrome.
- Those with other impaired absorption conditions, e.g. coeliacs or gastrectomy patients.

Therapeutic uses

- Vitamin A is used successfully in the treatment of certain skin conditions, e.g. acne and psoriasis.

——————————— SAFETY ———————————

Taken in excess, vitamin A can lead to toxicity because it is stored in the liver. However, it still has a high safety margin in that regular daily intakes generally have to exceed 7500mcg (25,000iu) in women, and 9000mcg (30,000iu) in men, before toxic side effects are experienced. The vitamin A intake of pregnant women, or women likely to become pregnant, should not exceed 3300mcg (11,000iu) per day (combined from food and supplements) unless directed. The effects of vitamin A excess would take the form of skin scaling, joint pains, liver enlargement and nausea. Vitamin A toxicity is usually fully reversible.

INTERACTIONS AND CONTRAINDICATIONS

Vitamin A and vitamin D are found together in many food sources, although they are not actually dependent upon one another for their absorption or utilisation. A deficiency of the mineral zinc can affect the function of vitamin A and vice versa. Vitamin A should not be taken with vitamin A derivative acne drugs. The need for vitamin A is decreased if you are on the contraceptive pill.

---

bETA CAROTENE

Did you know?

- Beta carotene is found in the yellow or orange pigment present in many fruits and vegetables.
- The human body can readily convert beta carotene into vitamin A.
- In 1830 the yellow pigment in carrots was isolated and named carotene; however, it was not until 1919 that the connection between carotene and vitamin A was known.
- It is now known that people with high levels of beta carotene in their diets have less chance of developing certain types of cancers than those with a lower intake of the nutrient.

Benefits

- In addition to all the functions for vitamin A, beta carotene is thought to be a free radical quencher. This means it has the capacity to protect delicate cell contents from damage.

Deficiency symptoms

- Deficiency symptoms of beta carotene are the same as for vitamin A.

Measurement

- Ius of beta carotene should not be confused with ius of

vitamin A activity. (Only ius of vitamin A have scientific meaning.) Ius of beta carotene divided by three gives ius of vitamin A activity, so a traditionally labelled 25,000iu (15mg) beta carotene supplement will provide the body with 8333iu of vitamin A.

Requirements (RNI)

- As dietary beta carotene contributes towards total vitamin A intake, there is no separate requirement for beta carotene.

Best Food Sources

Food	Beta carotene providing vitamin A (mcg/100g)	(iu/100g)	Food	Beta carotene providing vitamin A (mcg/100g)	(iu/100g)
Carrots (old)	12000	6667	Mango	1200	667
Spinach	6000	3333	Tomatoes	600	333
Sweet potato	4000	2233	Cabbage	300	167
Apricots, dried	3600	2000	Peas, frozen	300	167
Watercress	3000	1667	Potatoes	0	0

Who may need to supplement

- Many studies now show that low intakes of beta carotene are associated with the development of cancer and heart disease. With this in mind, nutrition experts underline the importance of taking two to three good portions of fruit and vegetables daily. If this sort of dietary level is not being achieved, a supplement of beta carotene may be advisable.
- Beta carotene supplementation is also recommended before prolonged exposure to hot sun. It can help to protect the skin from ultraviolet induced damage and may even protect against skin cancer in the long term.

N.B. The Medicines Act 1968 strictly prohibits any product being recommended for cancer treatment.

SAFETY

Beta carotene is an extremely safe form of taking vitamin A, because at very high levels of beta carotene intake, the body's beta carotene-to-vitamin A conversion process slows down dramatically.

The only known side effect occurring with high levels of beta carotene is 'carotenaemia', a harmless condition in which the skin turns a slight orange colour. This is reversible upon stopping beta carotene supplementation. Carotenaemia may occur at dosages of approximately 30mg daily and above.

INTERACTIONS AND CONTRAINDICATIONS

Beta carotene cannot be properly converted into vitamin A by diabetics or those with hypothyroidism or severe liver malfunctioning. These people should therefore not rely on beta carotene as a source of vitamin A activity.

THE *b* VITAMINS

Did you know?

- There are eight different B vitamins that work better together (synergistically) than as separate vitamins. This is why the B vitamins are referred to as B-complex.
- All the B-complex vitamins are water soluble, so a daily intake is vital.
- The B-complex vitamins are:

  Thiamin (B1);   Pyridoxine (B6);
  Riboflavin (B2);   Biotin;
  Niacin (B3);   Folic acid;
  Pantothenic acid (B5); Cobalamin (B12).

tHIAMIN (B1)

Did you know?

- Thiamin is known as the 'morale vitamin' because of the beneficial effects it has on the nervous system and morale.
- People with a low level of thiamin seem to be troubled more by insects.
- People with heart disease have been found to have lower than normal levels of thiamin in their heart muscle.
- Beriberi was found to be preventable if whole brown rice was eaten – in 1926 two doctors isolated the active ingredient, which turned out to be thiamin.
- Thiamin is very delicate and destroyed easily – after vitamin C, it is the least stable vitamin.
- Alcohol destroys thiamin.

Benefits

- Thiamin ensures mental alertness.
- It is vital for the release of energy from carbohydrates, fats and alcohol.
- During pregnancy, thiamin ensures the correct growth of the foetus.
- Thiamin ensures good digestion.

Deficiency symptoms

- Severe deficiency is now extremely rare in the West, but very low intakes lead to beriberi; symptoms of this are muscle weakness, nausea, loss of appetite and water retention.
- Minor deficiency will lead to mental problems, such as loss of concentration, depression, irritability and memory loss. Weight loss and digestive upsets also occur.
- Probably the earliest symptom of deficiency is continuous nausea.

Measurement

- Mg (milligrams).

Requirements (RNI)

THE RNI VALUES (COMA 1991) FOR THIAMIN			
Age	**(mg/day)**	**Age**	**(mg/day)**
0–9 months	0.2	15–18 years (males)	1.1
10–12 months	0.3	15+ years (females)	0.8
1–3 years	0.5	19–50 years (males)	1.0
4–10 years	0.7	50+ years (males)	0.9
11–14 years (females)	0.7	Pregnancy (last trimester)	0.9
11–14 years (males)	0.9	Lactation	1.0

Best Food Sources

Food	Thiamin (mg/100g)	Food	Thiamin (mg/100g)
Yeast extract	3.1	Peanuts, roasted	0.23
Fortified breakfast cereal	1.8	Bread, white	0.21
Soya beans, dry	1.10	Potatoes	0.2
Pork chop	0.57	Chicken	0.11
Rice	0.41	Beef, stewing steak	0.06
Bread, wholemeal	0.34	Milk	0.05
Peas, frozen	0.32		

Who may need to supplement

- The elderly.
- Pregnant women.
- Smokers.
- Alcoholics.
- People under physical or mental stress.
- People who have a high carbohydrate intake.
- Convalescents from surgery or accident.

Therapeutic uses

- Sciactica.
- Lumbago.
- Deters insect bites.

SAFETY

Thiamin is a very safe vitamin. Long-term, high amounts can be taken orally by adults without problems. Allergic reactions do sometimes arise when thiamin is injected into the body.

INTERACTIONS AND CONTRAINDICATIONS

Thiamin acts with the other B-complex vitamins, but can be taken on its own as part of nutritional therapy.

---

*R*IBOFLAVIN (B2)

Did you know?

- Riboflavin has a yellow colour and as a result has been used as a food colouring.
- Riboflavin is water soluble, so a regular daily intake is vital.
- It is very sensitive to light, so a pint of milk standing on the doorstep in the sunlight will lose almost all its vitamin B2 content.

Benefits

- Riboflavin forms two essential co-enzymes, (flavin dinuleotide and flavin mononumleotide) which together are responsible for converting proteins, fats and sugars into substances that the body can use.
- Riboflavin is important for healthy skin and hair.

Deficiency symptoms

- Cold sores.
- Burning, itchy eyes that tire easily and are sensitive to light.
- Dermatitis.
- Hair loss.

Measurement

- Mg (milligrams).

Requirements (RNI)

THE RNI VALUES (COMA 1991) FOR RIBOFLAVIN			
Age	(mg/day)	Age	(mg/day)
0–12 months	0.4	11+ years (females)	1.1
1–3 years	0.6	15+ years (males)	1.3
4–6 years	0.8	Pregnancy	1.4
7–10 years	1.0	Lactation	1.6
11–14 years (males)	1.2		

Best food sources

Food	Riboflavin (mg/100g)	Food	Riboflavin (mg/100g)
Yeast extract	11.0	Cheese, cheddar	0.5
Lamb's liver	4.64	Eggs	0.47
Pig's kidney	2.58	Beef, stewing steak	0.23
Fortified breakfast cereal	1.6	Milk	0.17
Wheatgerm	0.61	Chicken	0.13

Who may need to supplement

- Women on the contraceptive pill.
- Adults with irregular or poor eating habits.
- Vegetarians and vegans.

Therapeutic uses

- For sores and ulcers.
- For eye problems.
- For migraines (although there is no explanation for this).
- For muscle cramps.

————————————————— **SAFETY** —————————————————

Riboflavin is a safe vitamin, and no cases of riboflavin poisoning have ever been recorded.

INTERACTIONS AND CONTRAINDICATIONS

Riboflavin is one of the B-complex vitamins and works best when taken with the other B vitamins. However, it can be taken on its own for specific nutritional therapy; in this case it should be taken with brewer's yeast. Riboflavin can sometimes cause a harmless yellow colouring of the urine.

ℕIACIN (B3)

Did you know?

- Niacin comes in two forms: acid (nicotinic acid) and amide (nicotinamide) – neither of which has anything in common with nicotine.
- Niacin was also referred to as 'PP' because it prevented pellagra, a niacin deficiency disease whose symptoms are diarrhoea, dermatitis and dementia.
- In common with the other B vitamins, niacin is water soluble.
- In addition to preformed niacin occuring in foods, niacin may also be made in the body from an amino acid called tryptophan. Sixty molecules of tryptophan are required to make one molecule of niacin.

Benefits

- The acid form, nicotinic acid, plays an important role in the nervous system and circulation.
- The amide form, nicotinamide, processes carbohydrates, fats and protein as part of the production of energy.

Deficiency symptoms

- Diarrhoea, dermatitis and dementia (pellagra).
- Nervous tension.

Measurement

- Mg (milligrams).

Requirements (RNI)

THE RNI VALUES (COMA 1991) FOR NIACIN			
Age	(mg/day)	Age	(mg/day)
0–6 months	3	15–18 years (females)	14
7–9 months	4	15–18 years (males)	18
10–12 months	5	19–50 years (females)	13
1–3 years	8	19–50 years (males)	17
4–6 years	11	50+ years (females)	12
7–10 years	12	50+ years (males)	16
11–14 years (females)	12	Lactation	15
11–14 years (males)	15		

Best food sources

Food	Niacin (mg/100g)	Tryptophan (mg/100g)	Niacin equiv. (mg/100g)
Coffee, instant	24.8	186	27.9
Chicken	5.9	221	9.6
Beef, stewing steak	4.2	258	8.5
Pork chop	4.2	180	7.2
Cheese, Cheddar	0.1	367	6.2
Fish, white	2.9	189	6.0
Mung beans, dry	2.0	210	5.5
Eggs	0.1	217	3.7
Peas, frozen	1.6	58	2.6
Bread, wholemeal	4.1*	108	1.8
Potatoes	0.6	52	1.5

The niacin in wholemeal bread is unavailable to the body; the niacin equivalent figure comes from the tryptophan contribution.

Who may need to supplement

- Schizophrenics.
- Alcoholics.

Therapeutic uses

- Arthritis sufferers have found niacin supplementation can improve mobility.
- Alcoholics demonstrate the same type of mental disturbance as schizophrenics, and both groups respond better to niacin supplementation in megadoses (strictly under medical supervision) than to many drug treatments.
- Under medical supervision, megadoses of niacin have been known to reduce blood cholesterol.

--- **SAFETY** ---

Nicotinic acid can cause flushing if taken in megadoses. The Health Food Manufacturers' Association recommends as a result that timed-release nicotinic acid should not be available, and the maximum dosage should be 100mg. Nicotinamide is considered safe up to 2000mg/day.

INTERACTIONS AND CONTRAINDICATIONS

Niacin works with the other B-complex vitamins, but may be taken separately as part of nutritional therapy. If taken singly, it should be combined with thiamin and pyridoxine which taken together ensure nervous stability and the conversion of L-tryptophan to nicotinic acid. People suffering from diabetes, gout, stomach ulcers and liver problems should not take nicotinic acid.

$\mathcal{P}$ANTOTHENIC ACID (B5)

Did you know?

- Pantothenic acid, B5, is known as B3 in parts of Europe.
- Its name comes from the Greek *panthos*, which means 'everywhere'. Pantothenic acid is widely found everywhere – in our body tissues and in plants.
- Pantothenic acid is water soluble, so a regular daily intake is vital.
- It was first isolated from rice husks in 1939.

Benefits

- Pantothenic acid is very important to the process of releasing energy from foods. This is because it is part of coenzyme A, which plays a major role in energy release.
- Pantothenic acid is used to make and renew our body tissues.
- It is vital for the production of antibodies (part of our immune system).

Deficiency symptoms

- Tiredness.
- Depression.
- Loss of appetite.
- Cramps.
- Indigestion.
- Insomnia.

Measurement

- Mg (milligrams).

Requirements (RNI)

The COMA report of 1991 does not give specific recommended intakes of pantothenic acid because there is no standard to measure how much is already in the body (factors such as intestinal bacteria, length and usage of antibiotics, and so on, all play a part). However, an average of 3–7mg daily is thought to be sufficient for most adults.

Best food sources

Food	Pantothenic Acid (mg/100g)	Food	Pantothenic Acid (mg/100g)
Brewer's yeast	9.5	Wheat bran	2.4
Pig's liver	6.5	Wheatgerm	2.2
Yeast extract	3.8	Eggs	1.8
Nuts	2.7	Poultry	1.2

Who may need to supplement

- Alcoholics.
- Women on the contraceptive pill.
- Pregnant women.
- Smokers.

Therapeutic uses

- Relieves nausea.
- Relieves PMS.
- Treats 'burning feet' syndrome.
- Skin disorders.

———————————— SAFETY ————————————

Pantothenic acid is not recorded to date as being toxic.

INTERACTIONS AND CONTRAINDICATIONS

As one of the B-complex vitamins, pantothenic acid works best when taken as part of the complex, although it can be taken on its own as part of nutritional therapy.

It is linked with riboflavin in its function of energy production.

*P*YRIDOXINE (B6)

Did you know?

- Pyridoxine is known as the 'women's vitamin' because it is particularly beneficial for women.
- Pyridoxine is water soluble, so a regular daily intake is vital.
- Pyridoxine is essential to produce adrenalin and insulin.
- It is reasonably resistant to heat, but will leach out into water.
- High protein diets increase the need for pyridoxine.
- Alcoholics have low levels of pyridoxine.

Benefits

- Pyridoxine is essential for energy production
- It is vital for the nervous system.
- Pyridoxine is involved in protein metabolism.

Deficiency symptoms

- PMS.
- Seborrhoea (oily skin with crusts and scales) around the eyes, nose and mouth.
- Lowered white blood cell count.
- Swollen ankles, abdomen and fingers.

Measurement

- Mg (milligrams).

Requirements (RNI)

THE RNI VALUES (COMA 1991) FOR PYRIDOXINE*			
Age	(mg/day)	Age	(mg/day)
0–6 months	0.2	7–10 years	1.0
7–9 months	0.3	11–14 years (males)	1.2
10–12 months	0.4	11+ years (female)	1.0
1–3 years	0.7	15–18 years (males)	1.5
4–6 years	0.9	19+ years (males)	1.4

* Based on protein intake that provides 14.7% of average energy intake.

Best food sources

Food	Vitamin B6 (mg/100g)	Food	Vitamin B6 (mg/100g)
Wheatgerm	0.95	Potatoes	0.25
Bananas	0.51	Bread, wholemeal	0.12
Turkey	0.44	Baked beans	0.12
Chicken	0.29	Peas, frozen	0.10
Fish, white	0.29	Bread, white	0.07
Beef, stewing steak	0.27	Oranges	0.06
Brussels sprouts	0.28	Milk	0.06

Who may need to supplement

- Women on the contraceptive pill.
- Alcoholics.
- Lactating women.
- Smokers.
- People with heart disease.
- Women following hormone replacement therapy.

Therapeutic uses

- Cystitis.
- 'Flu.
- Conjunctivitis.

SAFETY

Pyridoxine is very safe to take, with no reported cases of toxicity. However, doses in excess of 100mg daily should be under strict medical supervision.

INTERACTIONS AND CONTRAINDICATIONS

Pyridoxine is one of the B-complex vitamins and so ideally should be taken as part of the complex, although single supplementation is acceptable as part of nutritional therapy.

COBALAMIN (B12)

Did you know?

- Vegans and vegetarians are likely to be short of cobalamin because it is available in meat products and is not normally found in vegetables.
- Cobalamin was the last true vitamin to be classified.

Benefits

- Cobalamin maintains a healthy nervous system.
- It promotes growth in children.
- It is needed for production of red blood cells.
- Cobalamin maintains the protective 'myelin sheath' around the nerves.
- Cobalamin is used to metabolise fatty acids.

Deficiency symptoms

- Pernicious anaemia, i.e. a shortfall of red blood cells. Note: if enough folic acid is taken, the symptoms of pernicious anaemia are hidden until irreversible neurological damage is done.
- Menstrual problems.
- Listlessness.
- Tremors.

Measurement

- Mcg (micrograms)

Requirements (RNI)

THE RNI VALUES (COMA 1991) FOR COBALAMIN			
Age	(mcg/day)	Age	(mcg/day)
0–6 months	0.3	7–10 years	1.0
7–12 months	0.4	11–14 years	1.2
1–3 years	0.5	15+ years	1.5
4–6 years	0.8	Lactation	2.0

Best food sources

Food	Vitamin B12 (mcg/100g)	Food	Vitamin B12 (mcg/100g)
Lamb's liver	54.0	Fortified breakfast cereal	1.7
Pig's liver	23.0	Eggs	1.7
Fish, white	2.0	Yeast extract	0.5
Beef, lamb, pork	2.0	Milk	0.4

Who may need to supplement

- Vegans and vegetarians.
- Alcoholics.
- Pregnant women.
- The elderly.
- Smokers.
- People who take medicines for stomach ulcers and similar conditions.

Therapeutic uses

- People suffering from moodiness and paranoia respond positively to cobalamin.
- It can provide relief from symptoms such as mental fatigue and memory impairment.
- Cobalamin detoxifies chemicals in tobacco smoke.

--- **SAFETY** ---

Cobalamin is a very safe vitamin, with injections of 3mg daily carried out with no side effects.

INTERACTIONS AND CONTRAINDICATIONS

Cobalamin is part of the B-complex and therefore works best synergistically. However, single supplementation of cobalamin is safe for specific nutritional therapy.

Calcium is required to absorb cobalamin from the bowel.

*f*OLIC ACID

Did you know?

- A study showed that 93 per cent of men and 98 per cent of women (aged 18–54) and 84 per cent of women aged over 55 in this country are deficient in folic acid.
- Up to 65 per cent of folic acid is lost during cooking.
- Folic acid was so named because it is found in green leaves, or foliage.
- Folic acid is water soluble and sensitive to light, heat and air.
- Low folic acid intake is associated with spina bifida.
- Women intending to start a family are now advised to supplement with folic acid before getting pregnant.

Benefits

- Folic acid is involved in passing on the genetic code to offspring.
- It is also involved in the formation of healthy cells.
- Folic acid is needed for DNA production and cell division.

Deficiency symptoms

- Anaemia, for which symptoms are: weakness, insomnia, forgetfulness, mental confusion and breathlessness.

Measurement

- Mcg (micrograms).

Requirements (RNI)

THE RNI VALUES (COMA 1991) FOR FOLIC ACID			
Age	(mcg/day)	Age	(mcg/day)
0–12 months	50	11+ years	200
1–3 years	70	Pregnancy	300
4–6 years	100	Lactation	260
7–10 years	150		

Best food sources

Food	Folic acid (mcg/100g)	Food	Folic acid (mcg/100g)
Brewer's yeast	2400	Bread, wholemeal	39
Wheatgerm	310	Eggs	30
Wheat bran	260	Bread, white	27
Nuts	110	Fish, fatty	26
Pig's Liver	110	Bananas	22
Leafy green vegetables	90	Potatoes	14
Pulses	80		

Who may need to supplement

- Pregnant women, because the foetus makes large demands on the folic acid stores.
- Coeliacs.
- The elderly, who tend to have poorer diets or impaired absorption.
- Alcoholics.

Therapeutic uses

- Folic acid supplements must be used under medical supervision for the treatment of megaloblastic anaemia, as folic acid can mask a vitamin B12 deficiency.

SAFETY

Folic acid is generally regarded as low risk, but megadoses are to be avoided (15mg per day). For this reason high dosages are not available.

INTERACTIONS AND CONTRAINDICATIONS

As one of the B-complex vitamins, folic acid is best taken as part of the complex.

*b*IOTIN

Did you know?

- Biotin, a water-soluble member of the B-complex, is sometimes referred to as 'vitamin H' or 'coenzyme R'.
- It was first discovered as a factor that protected against the toxicity of raw egg whites.

Benefits

- Biotin is required to process carbohydrates, energy and fats.
- Biotin prevents premature greying and balding.

Deficiency symptoms

- Scaly dermatitis occurs in adults, also known as cradle cap when infants suffer with the same complaint.
- Hair loss.
- Biotin deficiency is more common in babies than in adults.

Measurements

- Mcg (micrograms).

Requirements (RNI)

The COMA report suggests intakes of 10–200mcg. The band is wide because not enough is yet known about biotin. Actual intakes have been found to lie between 10 and 58mcg daily.

Best food sources

Food	Biotin (mcg/100g)	Food	Biotin (mcg/100g)
Brewer's yeast	80	Wheatgerm	12
Pig's kidney	32	Chicken`	10
Yeast extract	27	Lamb	6
Pig's liver	27	Bread, wholemeal	6
Wheat bran	14	Fish, fatty	5

Who may need to supplement

- Infants suffering from dermatitis and Leiner's disease.
- Pregnant women.

Therapeutic uses

- Treats cradle cap.
- Alleviates dermatitis and eczema.
- Is thought to relieve Candida albicans.

--- SAFETY ---

Having been given to young babies at dosages up to 40mg without problems, biotin is regarded as a safe vitamin.

INTERACTIONS AND CONTRAINDICATIONS

Biotin, as part of the B-complex, is best taken as part of the group of B vitamins, although single supplementation is safe as part of nutritional therapy.

*C*HOLINE AND INOSITOL

Did you know?

- Choline and inositol, members of the B-complex, are both found inside our bodies' cell walls.
- Choline increases the production of lecithin, which in turn breaks down fats.
- Inositol plays a part in the response of the nerve impulses.
- Inositol is found in large amounts in semen and men's reproductive organs.
- Inositol is not a true vitamin, because our bodies can make a small amount of it.

Benefits

- Inositol prevents eczema.
- Inositol has been shown to reduce irritability and stress levels.
- Choline helps to control cholesterol.

Deficiency symptoms

- Senile dementia.
- Eczema.
- High blood pressure.
- Nervousness.
- Reduced immune system – picking up every cold and cough that is going around.

Measurement

- Mg (milligrams)

Requirements (RNI)

- It is recommended that somewhere in the region of 500–1000mg of both choline and inositol is taken in on a daily basis.

Best food sources

Food	Choline (mg/100g)	Inositol (mg/100g)	Food	Choline (mg/100g)	Inositol (mg/100g)
Liver, dessicated	2170	1100	Nuts	220	180
Heart, beef	1720	1600	Pulses	120	160
Liver	650	340	Citrus fruits	85	210
Beef, steak	600	260	Bread, wholemeal	80	100
Brewer's yeast	300	50	Bananas	44	120

Who may need to supplement

- People with high cholesterol and/or hardening arteries.
- People with eczema.
- People suffering from stress and tension.

Therapeutic uses

- Choline improves our resistance to disease.
- Inositol strengthens the nervous system.
- Choline can improve angina and thrombosis when taken as lecithin.

SAFETY

Both choline and inositol are generally safe to take, although high doses (several grams per day) have been connected with resulting depression.

INTERACTIONS AND CONTRAINDICATIONS

None has been recorded for either inositol or choline.

$\mathcal{P}$ ABA

Did you know?

- The full name of PABA is: Para-aminobenzoic acid.
- PABA is the newest addition to the B-complex group, and strictly speaking is not a true vitamin, but a part of folic acid.
- PABA is essential for friendly bacteria to grow.
- PABA is recognised as having a cosmetic value, because it can stop hair turning grey.

Benefits

- The role of PABA is not yet fully explored, but it is thought to be helpful for:
  - the metabolism of red blood cells and amino acids.
  - a healthy skin.

Deficiency symptoms

- Because the action of PABA is not yet fully known, deficiency symptoms are also not known.

Measurement

- G (grams)

Requirements (RNI)

- As yet there are no official guidelines regarding a daily intake of PABA.

Best food sources

Not many figures are produced on the amount of PABA in food. However, liver, eggs, wheatgerm and molasses are known to be good sources.

Therapeutic uses

- Major accepted use of PABA is as a remedy for vitiligo (a condition characterised by de-pigmentation of the skin).
- PABA has been used in sclerodoma (thickening of the skin) and in lupus erythematosus – another severe skin disorder. However, the dosages used in clinical trials for these conditions were extremely high and should not be self-administered.

— SAFETY —

PABA is best taken with the other B vitamins but can be taken on its own if required. Dosages in excess of 8g daily may result in constant itching and, more seriously, liver complaints.

INTERACTIONS AND CONTRAINDICATIONS

None has been recorded to date.

$\mathcal{V}$ITAMIN C

Did you know?

- Vitamin C is also known as 'ascorbic acid' – the name which appears on food labels.
- Humans, guinea-pigs, apes and the Indian fruit bat are the only species on our planet that cannot make vitamin C: as a result we rely on our food and drink to supply us with this vitamin.
- In 1768 James Lind formally noted that eating citrus fruits warded off scurvy. As a result, English sailors used to carry limes on board to prevent scurvy – which led to their nickname 'limeys'.
- Vitamin C is very delicate: it is water soluble, and sensitive to heat, air and light. Our bodies cannot store it so a regular daily intake is vital.
- Smoking depletes vitamin C, so smokers need a higher daily intake than non-smokers.

Benefits

- Vitamin C is involved in over 300 biological processes, which explains why it is so important.
- It is important for the immune system to function effectively.
- Vitamin C is used to make collagen – the body's intercellular 'cement'.
- It speeds up the healing of wounds and torn tissue, and ensures growth.
- Vitamin C helps the body to absorb iron properly, and to breakdown folic acid in a form which the body can use.

Deficiency symptoms

- Signs of scurvy are usually first to be observed, and these include: bleeding gums; muscle and joint aches and pains; dry, scaly skin; irritability; easy bruising.
- Prolonged marginal deficiency may predispose towards cancer and heart disease.

Measurements

- Mg (milligrams)

Requirements (RNI)

THE RNI VALUES (COMA 1991) FOR VITAMIN C			
Age	(mg/day)	Age	(mg/day)
0–12 months	25	15+ years	40
1–10 years	30	Pregnancy	50
11–14 years	35	Lactation	70

Best food sources

- Potatoes, fruit juice, citrus fruit and green vegetables.

Food	Vitamin C (mg/100g)	Food	Vitamin C (mg/100g)
Blackcurrants	200	Tomatoes	20
Pepper, green	100	Potatoes	
Brussels sprouts	90	new	16
Mango	80	Oct–Dec	19
Cauliflower	60	Jan–Feb	9
Cabbage	55	Mar–May	8
Oranges	50	Lettuce	15
Grapefruit	40	Bananas	10
Sweet potatoes	25		

Who may need to supplement

- The elderly.
- The ill.
- Pregnant or lactating women.
- Athletes.
- Smokers.
- People who drink a lot of alcohol.
- People regularly taking antibiotics, aspirin, the contraceptive pill and steroids.
- Those who have recurrent infection.

Therapeutic uses

- Colds and 'flu.
- Prior to and post dental treatment.
- Stress relief.
- Alcoholism.
- Toxic poisoning.
- Osteoarthritis.

──────────────── **SAFETY** ────────────────

People with kidney stones should avoid high dosages of vitamin C ('high' being over 1g daily). If you take very high doses (in excess of 5000mg) daily, do not stop the dosage suddenly, but reduce the amount gradually.

Otherwise, this is a very safe vitamin and the body easily expels excesses. Mild diarrhoea may result if the body is trying to rid itself of excessively large amounts of unwanted vitamin C.

INTERACTIONS AND CONTRAINDICATIONS

Bioflavinoids increase the activity of vitamin C; they always appear naturally with vitamin C. They are stable, unlike vitamin C, and increase its absorption.

High levels of vitamin C will push up the requirement for calcium.

Vitamin C is one of the antioxidant nutrients (vitamins A, C and E, and minerals zinc and selenium).

Vitamin C may dilute anti-depressants (tricyclic).

$\mathcal{V}$ITAMIN D

Did you know?

- Vitamin D is called the 'sunshine vitamin'.
- There are two types of vitamin D:
  Cholecalciferol (vitamin D3) found in animal liver oils, and the effect of sunlight on cholesterol deposits in the skin; and *Ergocalciferol* (vitamin D2) which is produced when ultra-violet light affects the precursor ergosterol (the 'vegetarian' form of vitamin D).
- In the seventeenth century, the smog and naturally dull English weather caused many children to have rickets (twisted, malformed limbs). Rickets became known as 'the English disease'.
- Children need more vitamin D than adults.
- Vitamin D is stored in the liver and is fat soluble.

Benefits

- The most important role played by vitamin D is in bone development. It works by being converted to a hormone which itself controls calcium absorption which again in turn affects bone development. This is why children have a higher requirement of vitamin D than adults.
- Vitamin D is essential for the development of strong, healthy teeth.

Deficiency Symptoms

- The adult version of rickets is osteomalacia, for which symptoms include brittle bones, bone pain and muscular spasms.
- In children, knock-knees are the most evident sign of vitamin D deficiency.
- Children may be late in growing teeth.
- Children grow with an unnatural posture.

Measurement

- Mcg and ius. Conversion factor is 1iu to 40mcg.

Requirements (RNI)

THE RNI VALUES (COMA 1991) FOR VITAMIN D					
Age	(mcg/day)	(iu/day)	Age	(mcg/day)	(iu/day)
0–6 months	8.5	340	Pregnancy	10	400
7 months–3 years	7.0	280	Lactation	10	400

It was decided by the COMA panel that in the 3 to 65 year age group, vitamin D formed from skin exposure to the sun was usually sufficient to satisfy needs, and that an extra dietary supply was therefore generally unnecessary.

Best food sources

Food	Vitamin D (mcg/100g)	(iu/100g)	Food	Vitamin D (mcg/100g)	(iu/100g)
Cod liver oil	212.5	8500	Butter	0.8	32
Herring and kipper	22.4	896	Liver	0.8	32
Salmon, canned	12.5	500	Cheese, cheddar	0.3	12
Milk, evaporated	4.0	160	Milk, whole	0.03	1.2
Eggs	1.6	64	Milk, skimmed	0	0

Who may need to supplement

- Vegetarians and vegans, because vitamin D is mostly in animal products.
- Asian immigrants, since their national dress prevents exposure to the sun's rays.
- Elderly or housebound people, who are also unlikely to have sufficient exposure to the sun
- Women who have had a series of pregnancies and as a result become short of calcium.
- Breast-feeding women whose milk may be short of vitamin D, especially during winter.

Therapeutic uses

- Treats rickets, (a deficiency of vitamin D leads to development of rickets).
- Strengthens bones and teeth.

────────────── **SAFETY** ──────────────

Vitamin D can be the most toxic of all the vitamins, so care must be taken not to exceed the recommended guidelines. However, vitamin D is safe up to five times the recommended amount. Too much vitamin D will affect the kidneys, heart and lungs.

INTERACTIONS AND CONTRAINDICATIONS

Vitamin D is important for the absorption of calcium and phosphate.

Although vitamins A and D are often found together, they are not, in fact, co-dependent.

Some cardiac drugs when taken with vitamin D may cause irregular heart rhythm, so consult your doctor if this is likely to affect you.

$\mathcal{V}$ITAMIN E (TOCOPHEROL)

Did you know?

- This vitamin is one of the antioxidant nutrients (the others are vitamins A and C and the minerals selenium and zinc).
- Vitamin E is very good for the skin
- Vitamin E has had many names, one of the earliest was 'the anti-sterility vitamin'.
- Vitamin E is used to treat menopausal hot flushes, because it regulates the body's temperature.
- Vitamin E exists naturally in many different forms, and different strengths.

Benefits

- Vitamin E is a powerful antioxidant.
- It breaks down fats.
- It gives energy.
- Vitamin E protects the body's cells and other important nutrients.
- It aids healing.
- It prevents thrombosis.
- Vitamin E increases the efficiency of oxygen, so it can increase levels of fitness.
- Vitamin E is an anti-clotting agent.
- It is vital for the nervous system to function correctly.

Deficiency symptoms

- Deficiency of vitamin E is unlikely as it is easily and widely available, and if fats and oils can be absorbed there is no problem.
- There is no specific disease to show vitamin E deficiency, but chronic shortage of this vitamin is thought to lead to a host of illnesses, while some conditions are acknowledged to lead to a shortage of vitamin E. Such conditions include:
  - low red blood cell count, cirrhosis of the liver, alcoholism, coeliac disease, cystic fibrosis.

Measurement

- Iu and mg.

Requirements (RNI)

- The amount of vitamin E required is dependent upon the amount of PUFAs (polyunsaturated fatty acids) in the diet. The COMA 1991 report decided that the amount of PUFAs vary so much from person to person, as do individual requirements of vitamin E, that a fixed recommended amount was impossible to arrive at. However, 0.4mg/g PUFA has been judged suitable in the USA. If PUFAs provide 6 per cent of dietary energy, men would require 7mg per day and women 5mg per day.

Best food sources

Food	Vitamin E (mg/100g)	Food	Vitamin E (mg/100g)
Wheatgerm oil	178	Peanut butter	9
Safflower oil	97	Soybean oil	8
Sunflower seeds, raw	74	Butter	3
Sunflower oil	73	Asparagus	2.7
Almonds	37	Spinach	2.7
Mayonnaise	19	Broccoli	0.7
Wheatgerm	17	Bananas	0.3
Margarine, hard	16	Strawberries	0.3

Who may need to supplement

- Sufferers of Parkinson's disease.
- Those people with cardiovascular problems.

Therapeutic uses

- Women with menstrual or menopausal problems.
- People after undergoing surgery, to speed healing.
- People with poor circulation, varicose veins.

───────────────── **SAFETY** ─────────────────

Vitamin E is thought to be safe up to amounts of 3200 mg per day. Levels over 800 iu have occasionally been associated with fatigue, nausea, raised blood pressure and mild gastro-intestinal problems. These symptoms are reversible when a gradual decrease of intake is effected.

INTERACTIONS AND CONTRAINDICATIONS

If you are taking anticoagulant medicines, vitamin E must only be taken with your Doctor's approval.

Vitamin E activity is increased by selenium, and vice versa.

Diabetics are generally advised to avoid vitamin E supplements.

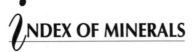

INDEX OF MINERALS

*b*ORON

Did you know?

- Boron is a mineral which is only essential for plants.
- Only recently has boron been recognised as playing a part in human nutrition. Its exact functions have yet to be discovered.

Benefits

- It is believed that boron is important to maintain bone density, and it is thought it may have particular relevance to women.
- Boron administered to menopausal women slowed the rate of calcium and magnesium losses and doubled levels of a compound, oestrogen metabolite, which is responsible for retaining calcium in the bone.
- Broken bones heal faster with boron supplementation.
- Rheumatoid arthritis symptoms diminish with boron supplementation.

Deficiency symptoms

- No specific symptoms have been recognised with regard to boron deficiency as yet, although a shortfall of boron in animals has been documented (stunted growth).

Measurement

- Mg (milligrams).

Requirements (RNI)

- Since boron has yet to be defined as essential for life, there is no RNI to date.

Best food sources

Food	Boron (mg/100g)	Food	Boron (mg/100g)
Soya	2.8	Peanuts	1.8
Prunes	2.7	Hazlenuts	1.6
Raisins	2.5	Dates	0.92
Almonds	2.3	Wine	up to 0.85
Rosehips	1.9	Honey	0.72

--- **SAFETY** ---

Boron is fatal when applied as boric acid externally: the body absorbs the boron in too large a quantity in this way. The situation is exacerbated if boron is applied to broken skin or membranes.

Vomiting and diarrhoea typically demonstrate boron toxicity.

Fatal doses are 15–20g, and in children 3–6g, but as little as 100mg may produce toxic effects. Short-term megadoses up to 9mg are usually safe, but take advice from your doctor.

INTERACTIONS AND CONTRAINDICATIONS

If boron is lost as a result of osteoporosis, extra calcium seems to make up for the loss.

Animal studies have shown that a deficiency of vitamin D increases the need for boron.

CALCIUM

Did you know?

- Calcium is the most abundant mineral in the human body: over 1.5 per cent of total body weight is calcium, found in the skeleton and tissues.
- To be absorbed, cobalamin (vitamin B12) needs calcium.
- Calcium needs vitamin D in order to be absorbed.
- We rely on our food and drink to supply us with calcium as our bodies cannot make it.
- Adults lose 400–600mg of calcium daily.

Benefits

- Calcium gives us strong bones and teeth.
- Calcium is required to ensure that blood clots correctly.
- Calcium found inside the body's cells transmits nerve impulses.
- Sufficient calcium intake will avoid osteoporosis in women aged over 35 years.

Deficiency symptoms

- Children will contract rickets.
- Menopausal women will contract osteroporosis.
- There is an increased susceptibility to bone fractures, particularly in the elderly.

Measurement

- Mg (milligrams).

Requirements (RNI)

THE RNI VALUES (COMA 1991) FOR CALCIUM			
Age	(mg/day)	Age	(mg/day)
0–12 months	525	11–18 years (males)	1000
1–3 years	350	11–18 years (females)	800
4–6 years	450	19+ years	700
7–10 years	550	Lactation	1250

Best food sources

Food	Calcium (mg/100g)	Food	Calcium (mg/100g)
Skimmed milk powder	1230	Natural yoghurt	200
Cheese, Cheddar	800	Milk	103
Sardines	550	Peanuts, roasted	61
Tofu	506	Cabbage	57
Dried figs	280	Bread, wholemeal	54
Evaporated milk	260	Eggs	52
Watercress	220	Fish, white	22

Who may need to supplement

- Pregnant and lactating women. Post-menopausal women.
- People who regularly take antacids.
- Vegans.

Therapeutic uses

- Calcium has been linked with periodontal disease and its treatment. Periodontal disease is when bone density reduces.
- Studies on people suffering from high blood pressure show improvement after taking calcium supplements.

——————————— SAFETY ———————————

Calcium is safe to take even in large amounts since the body rids itself of unwanted amounts.

INTERACTIONS AND CONTRAINDICATIONS

Calcium and vitamin D act together and calcium cannot be absorbed without sufficient vitamin D.

Calcium and magnesium, and calcium and potassium, seem to be related in that low levels of one produce high levels of the other.

Care must be taken to avoid excessive amounts of potassium which can lower calcium levels.

CHROMIUM

Did you know?

• As we age we retain less chromium.

Benefits

• Chromium breaks down sugar so that it can be used by the body: it is a deterrent to diabetes.
• Chromium maintains the correct blood pressure.

Deficiency symptoms

• High blood sugar levels.
• High cholesterol levels.
• Poor tolerance of glucose.

Measurement

• Mcg (micrograms).

Requirements (RNI)

• There is no RNI value for chromium as given by the COMA report, but a daily amount in excess of 25mcg is thought to be adequate and safe.

Best food sources

Food	Chromium (mg/100g)	Food	Chromium (mg/100g)
Egg yolk	183	Honey	29
Molasses	121	Potatoes, old	27
Brewer's yeast	117	Wheatgerm	23
Beef	57	Chicken leg	18
Cheese	56	Spaghetti	15
Grape juice	47	Spinach	10
Bread, wholemeal	42	Bananas	10
Wheat bran	38	Haddock	7
Raw sugar	35	Milk, skimmed	2

Who may need to supplement

- People tending towards diabetes.
- People wishing to lower cholesterol levels and increase HDL levels.

Therapeutic uses

- Athletes wishing to develop lean muscle.

INTERACTIONS AND CONTRAINDICATIONS

Chelated zinc has been found to be a good substitute for chromium.

COPPER

Did you know?

- Copper is used in contraceptive devices because it is toxic to sperm.
- 70 per cent of copper content is lost when flour is refined.
- Deficiency of dietary copper is thought to be responsible for increasing the risk of heart disease.

Benefits

- Copper is involved in many processes in our bodies, such as:
  - production of melanin, hence affecting the colour of our skin and hair;
  - the production of superoxide dismutase, a substance which protects us from free radicals and cell damage;
- Copper transmits nerve impulses to the brain.
- It is used in energy production.
- Copper is used in oxidising fatty acids.
- It is involved in transferring oxygen in the muscles.

Deficiency symptoms

- Babies lacking in copper have pale skin, diarrhoea and dilated veins.
- Adults lacking in copper develop anaemia.
- The white blood count falls in adults when there is a shortfall of copper.
- Sometimes the sense of taste fails.

Measurement

- Mg (milligrams).

Requirements (RNI)

THE RNI VALUES (COMA 1991) FOR COPPER			
Age	(mg/day)	Age	(mg/day)
9–12 months	0.3	11–14 years	0.8
1–3 years	0.4	15–16 years	1.0
4–6 years	0.6	18+ years	1.2
7–10 years	0.7	Lactation	1.5

Best food sources

Food	Copper (mg/100g)	Food	Copper (mg/100g)
Oysters	7.6	Hazlenuts	1.4
Whelks	7.2	Shrimps	0.8
Lamb's liver	6.0	Cod	0.6
Crab	4.8	Bread, wholemeal	0.25
Brewer's yeast	3.3	Peas	0.2
Olives	1.6		

Who may need to supplement

- If a zinc supplement is taken, a copper supplement may be needed since zinc depletes copper reserves.
- People with Menke's syndrome (a rare, genetic disease) need copper supplementation.

Therapeutic uses

- Alleviates arthritis symptoms.
- Relieves osteoarthritis symptoms.

SAFETY

Toxicity is rare, although this could be because copper supplementation as a single supplement is unusual. Regular intakes up to 10mg daily are safe but are advised not to be exceeded (FAO/WHO Expert Committee, 1971).

INTERACTIONS AND CONTRAINDICATIONS

Copper and zinc are linked, since zinc depletes copper.

Copper and vitamin A are linked, since vitamin A requires copper and other nutrients to be absorbed.

Vitamin C improves copper absorption.

---

*i*RON

Did you know?

- Iron is found in two different forms in food: haem iron is exclusive to animal, fish or birds, whilst non-haem iron is found in fruit and vegetables.
- The most common deficiency in all minerals and vitamins is of iron, the world over (World Health Organisation).
- Although iron is plentiful in the planet, and vital for humans, it exists in very small ('trace') amounts in our bodies – about 4–5g.

Benefits

- Iron is a vital ingredient of haemoglobin, the blood pigment.
- Iron is important in the production and release of energy.

- Iron helps to keep our immune systems working properly.
- Iron helps young children to grow physically and mentally.

Deficiency symptoms

- Tiredness, pale face, membrane in the eye is white instead of normal pink colour, fingernails no longer pink but white.
- If iron deficiency is allowed to progress past the above early symptoms, dizziness, fast pulse rate, loss of appetite and insomnia are experienced.
- Children short of iron will have stunted growth and their mental abilities will be damaged.
- Pruritis (generalised itching all over the body).

Measurement

- Mg (milligrams).

Requirements (RNI)

THE RNI VALUES (COMA 1991) FOR IRON			
Age	(mg/day)	Age	(mg/day)
0–3 months	1.7	7–10 years	8.7
4–6 months	4.3	11–18 years (males)	11.3
7–12 months	7.8	11–50 years (females)	14.8
1–3 years	6.9	19–50 years (males)	8.7
4–6 years	6.1	50+ years	8.7

Best food sources

Food	Iron (mg/100g)	Food	Iron (mg/100g)
Curry powder	29.6	Eggs	2.0
Fortified breakfast cereal	16.7	Beef	1.9
Lamb's liver	7.5	Watercress	1.6
Pig's kidney	6.4	Bread, white	1.6
Apricots, dried	4.1	Cabbage	0.6
Bread, wholemeal	2.7	Red wine	0.5
Corned beef	2.4	Fish, white	0.5
Chocolate, plain	2.4	Potatoes	0.4

Who may need to supplement

- Women of childbearing age, because of their monthly menstrual blood loss. Women with very heavy periods will need to increase their iron intake further.
- Vegetarians.
- The elderly.
- Pregnant women.
- Lactating women.
- Adolescents.
- Athletes.
- Alcoholics.

Therapeutic Uses

- Relieves pruritis.
- Treats mental disability in young children.
- Reverses problems caused by its deficiency.

--------------------------- SAFETY ---------------------------

Care needs to be taken with iron, since some people cannot tolerate large amounts, and children should not be given megadoses. Otherwise toxicity is not a common problem, and daily amounts of 25–75mg have been taken without side effects.

INTERACTIONS AND CONTRAINDICATIONS

Iron is best taken as part of an overall multi vitamin/mineral supplement.

Vitamin C improves absorption of haem iron (animal, fish or fowl origin). Copper is needed to turn iron into haemoglobin (used in the production of red blood cells).

$\mathcal{M}$AGNESIUM

Did you know?

- Magnesium is one of the most abundant minerals in the human body, following after calcium and phosphorous.
- Half of the body's magnesium is found in bones, the rest is in the body's tissues.
- Magnesium is vital for energy release.
- Magnesium is required to make DNA.
- Our muscles and nerves need magnesium to function properly.

Benefits

- Magnesium has a finger in almost every pie, biologically speaking. This means a shortfall of magnesium will have repercussions on just about every function of the body.
- Magnesium is essential for growth.
- It is used to keep the body's cells and tissues healthy.
- It keeps hormones working correctly.
- Magnesium is thought to have some protective effect on the heart.
- It is essential for nerve impulses.

Deficiency symptoms

- The nervous system is affected, leading to irritability, tension and stress.
- Muscle tremors and cramps.
- Frequent 'pins and needles'.
- Arrhythmia (irregular heartbeat).

Measurement

- Mg (milligrams).

Requirements (RNI)

THE RNI VALUES (COMA 1991) FOR MAGNESIUM			
Age	(mg/day)	Age	(mg/day)
0–3 months	55	7–10 years	200
4–6 months	60	11–14 years	280
7–9 months	75	15–18 years	300
10–12 months	80	19+ years (males)	300
1–3 years	85	19+ years (females)	270
4–6 years	120	Lactation	320

Best food sources

Food	Magnesium (mg/100g)	Food	Magnesium (mg/100g)
Peanuts, roasted	180	Beef, stewing steak	18
Bread, wholemeal	76	Potatoes	17
Cheese, cheddar	25	Oranges	13
Fish, white	23	Eggs	12
Chicken	21	Milk	10

Who may need to supplement

- Women suffering from PMS.
- Alcoholics.
- People taking diuretics.

Therapeutic uses

- Treats PMS.
- Relieves hyperactivity.
- Studies show that angina sufferers have benefitted from magnesium supplementation.

─────────── **SAFETY** ───────────

Magnesium is safe to take even in large doses, except for people with kidney problems.

ℳANGANESE

Did you know?

- Manganese is a trace mineral, which we cannot make ourselves but must obtain from our food and drink.
- 86 per cent of manganese content is lost when flour is refined.
- 89 per cent of manganese is lost when sugar is refined.
- Almost half of the UK's supply of manganese comes from drinking tea.

Benefits

- Manganese ensures our bones develop correctly and stay healthy.
- Manganese is present in women's sex hormones.
- A healthy nervous system requires manganese.

Deficiency symptoms

- Since manganese deficiency has only been observed in one person, it is impossible to describe the symptoms of manganese deficiency.
- However, in animals a shortfall of manganese results in problems with reproduction, stunted growth and deformed offspring.

Measurement

- Mg (milligrams).

Requirements (RNI)

- The COMA report does not give an RNI for manganese, but a safe intake is given at 'above 1.4mg daily for adults'.

Best Food Sources

Food	Manganese (mg/100g)	Food	Manganese (mg/100g)
Bread, wholemeal	4.3	Coconut	1.3
Wheatgerm	4.2	Pineapple	1.1
Avocados	4.2	Plums	1.0
Chestnuts	3.7	Lettuce	0.7
Hazelnuts	3.5	Bananas	0.6
Peas	2.0	Beetroot	0.6
Almonds	1.9	Watercress	0.5
Tea (1 cup)	1.5	Carrots	0.25

Who may need to supplement

- Non-tea drinkers!

SAFETY

Manganese supplements taken by mouth have not presented toxicity problems to date: inhaling dust from smelting works can be toxic, however.

Too much manganese in children has been associated with learning problems.

INTERACTIONS AND CONTRAINDICATIONS

Manganese is thought to increase the effects of iron when red blood cells are produced.

ℳOLYBDENUM

Did you know?

- Molybdenum is a trace mineral.

Benefits

- Xanthine oxidase is an enzyme responsible for iron metabolism and it requires molybdenum to function correctly.
- Molybdenum ensures normal sexual function in men.
- Uric acid is a waste product which is found in the blood and urine, and it needs molybdenum for its production.
- Excess copper is detoxified by molybdenum.

Deficiency symptoms

- Men experience problems with sexual functioning.

Measurement

- Mcg (micrograms).

Requirements (RNI)

The COMA report does not set an RNI for molybdenum, but states that a safe intake is 'between 50mcg and 400mcg'.

Best food sources

Food	Molybdenum (mcg/100g)	Food	Molybdenum (mcg/100g)
Canned beans	350	Eggs	50
Wheatgerm	200	Rice	47
Liver	200	Noodles	45
Lentils	120	Chicken	40
Sunflower seeds	103	Bread, wholemeal	26
Kidney	75	Potatoes	25
Green beans	66	Shell fish	20
Macaroni	51	Apricots	14

Who may need to supplement

- Those with proven molybdenum deficiency.
- People with excess blood copper levels.

Therapeutic uses

- None known for molybdenum.

--------------------------------- **SAFETY** ---------------------------------

Molybdenum is generally included in all-purpose multi vitamin/mineral supplements, so its toxicity levels as a separate supplement are not known to date by this author.

$\mathcal{P}$OTASSIUM

Did you know?

- Most of our potassium is inside the skeletal muscles, in the cells themselves.

Benefits

- The small amount of potassium that is outside our body cells helps to maintain normal blood pressure.
- The chief role of potassium is to maintain the correct amount of water in our cells.
- It helps to stabilise the structure of our body cells.
- Potassium maintains the acid–alkaline balance in our bodies.
- It stimulates the movements in the intestines.
- In partnership with sodium, potassium ensures the transmission of nerve impulses.

Deficiency Symptoms

- Listlessness.
- Loss of appetite and nausea.

- Thirst.
- Drowsiness.

Measurement

- Mg (milligrams).

Requirements (RNI)

THE RNI VALUES (COMA 1991) FOR POTASSIUM			
Age	(mg/day)	Age	(mg/day)
0–3 months	800	4–6 years	1100
4–6 months	850	7–10 years	2000
7–12 months	700	11–14 years	3100
1–3 years	800	15+ years	3500

Best food sources

Food	Potassium (mg/100g)	Sodium (mg/100g)
Instant coffee	3780	81
Potato crisps	1190	550
Raisins	860	52
Potatoes	360	8
Pork	360	65
Cauliflower	350	8
Tomatoes	290	3
Chicken	290	75
Bread, wholemeal	230	560
Peas, frozen	190	3
Streaky bacon	183	1245
Oranges	180	2
Milk, whole	140	50
Eggs	136	140
Cheese, Cheddar	120	610

Who may need to supplement

- People who take diuretics, since some diuretics deplete the body's amounts of potassium. Take medical advice first.

- Athletes or physical labourers who can lose potassium through sweat.
- People who are taking antibiotics on a long-term basis, since these can deplete stores of potassium.

Therapeutic uses

- People with high blood pressure.
- Relieves night cramps.

— **SAFETY** —

High intakes of potassium will cause problems in people with kidney complaints to the extent of having heart failure. Follow your doctor's advice if planning to take a separate supplement of potassium: generally it is better to take potassium as part of an overall multi vitamin/mineral supplement.

INTERACTIONS AND CONTRAINDICATIONS

Sodium and potassium combine to ensure the body has the correct water balance. A high salt intake will push up the requirement for potassium.

SELENIUM

Did you know?

- Selenium derives its name from the goddess of the moon, Selene.
- Selenium is an essential trace mineral and is only obtainable from our food and drink.
- Until 1979, it was thought that selenium was important only for animals, and a poison for humans. At this very late date, though, it was discovered that selenium is essential for humans.

- Selenium is 50 to 100 times more powerful an antioxidant than vitamin E.

Benefits

- Selenium is (like vitamins C and E) an antioxidant, so it destroys the potentially harmful free radicals.
- Selenium maintains a healthy heart and normal liver function.
- It also ensures eyes and eyesight function correctly.
- Healthy hair and skin depend on selenium.
- Selenium is thought to protect against cancer, in common with vitamins A, C and E and the mineral zinc.

Deficiency symptoms

- Selenium deficiency is fairly rare in the West while we continue to enjoy foods from other countries whose soil is still rich in selenium. For this reason specific deficiency symptoms relating to selenium are not documented. However, Keshan disease (a heart disease which primarily affects Chinese children) does arise when dietary intakes of selenium fall.

Measurement

- Mcg (micrograms).

Requirements (RNI)

THE RNI VALUES (COMA 1991) FOR SELENIUM			
Age	(mcg/day)	Age	(mcg/day)
0–3 months	10	11–14 years	45
4–6 months	13	15–18 years (males)	70
7–12 months	10	15+ years (females)	60
1–3 years	15	19+ years (males)	75
4–6 years	20	Lactation	75
7–10 years	30		

Best food sources

Food	Selenium (mcg/100g)	Food	Selenium (mcg/100g)
Organ meats*	approx. 40	Wholegrains and cereals	approx.12
Fish and shellfish	approx. 32	Dairy products	approx. 5
Meat	approx. 18	Fruit and vegetables	approx. 2

* Kidney, liver, muscle meats.

Who may need to supplement

- Young adults who may not be eating properly.
- Vegetarians.
- The elderly.
- Smokers.
- Pregnant women and nursing mothers.

Therapeutic uses

- Relieves arthritic symptoms.
- Lowers high blood pressure
- Improves skin, hair and nail problems.
- Detoxification of heavy metals (e.g. mercury in dental fillings).

——————————— **SAFETY** ———————————

Extremely high doses of selenium (5000mcg) taken over a long period of time have resulted in hair loss and deformed fingernails. Doses of 1000mcg over a long period have resulted in the sweat smelling of garlic despite the fact that no garlic was eaten, and thicker, but less strong fingernails. Diarrhoea, nausea, fatigue and irritability are other symptoms experienced by overdosing.

INTERACTIONS AND CONTRAINDICATIONS

Selenium works with vitamin E as an antioxidant and to relieve angina. Selenium in conjunction with vitamins C and E has inhibited cancer in laboratory studies with animals.

$\mathcal{V}$ANADIUM

- As yet not much is known about the role played by vanadium in our health.

Benefits

- Vanadium is needed for normal growth.
- This mineral plays a part in fertility.
- Lipid metabolism requires vanadium to function correctly.

Deficiency symptoms

- As yet not recorded.

Measurement

- Mcg (micrograms).

Requirements (RNI)

The COMA report does not list a recommended daily intake for vanadium, but since 10mcg is lost daily through urine, at least this amount is needed as a replacement.

Best food sources

Food	Vanadium (mcg/100g)	Food	Vanadium (mcg/100g)
Parsley	2950	Sardines	46
Lobster	1610	Cucumber	38
Radishes	790	Apples	33
Dill	460	Cauliflower	9
Lettuce	280	Tomatoes	4
Strawberries	70	Potatoes	1

—————————————— **SAFETY** ——————————————

Vanadium can easily be toxic if taken in synthetic form.

$\mathcal{Z}$INC

Did you know?

- Zinc is a trace mineral: only 2–3g are to be found in the adult body.
- Zinc is part of over 80 enzymes, which means that it has more functions than any other trace mineral.

Benefits

- Zinc keeps nails, skin and hair healthy.
- Zinc maintains the reproductive organs in both men and women.

Deficiency symptoms

- White flecks in the nails.
- Acne, eczema and psoriasis where these are caused by zinc deficiency.
- Lowered immune system – picking up all the infections going around.

Measurement

- Mg (milligrams).

Requirements (RNI)

THE RNI VALUES (COMA 1991) FOR ZINC			
Age	(mg/day)	Age	(mg/day)
0–6 months	4.0	15+ years (males)	9.5
7 months–3 years	5.0	15+ years (females)	7.0
4–6 years	6.5	Lactation (0–4 months)	13.0
7–10 years	7.0	(4+ months)	9.5
11–14 years	9.0		

Best Food Sources

Food	Zinc (mg/100g)	Food	Zinc (mg/100g)
Cheese, Cheddar	4.0	Bread, white	0.6
Beef, stewing steak	3.8	Milk	0.4
Bread, wholemeal	1.8	Fish, white	0.4
Eggs	1.5	Potatoes, old	0.3
Chicken	1.1		

Who may need to supplement

- Pregnant women, since the foetus needs zinc to develop.
- Vegetarians, because vegetables tend to bind the zinc which then is not absorbed by the body.

Therapeutic uses

- Sufferers of rheumatoid arthritis may find some improvement with zinc supplementation because zinc and essential fatty acids are interlinked.
- Treat prostate problems, or prevent them.
- Adolescents, to relieve acne.
- Sufferers of the common cold – zinc and vitamin C combined strengthen the immune system and so fight off the infection sooner.

SAFETY

Megadoses of zinc (150–450mg daily) have been shown to cause low white blood cell count and small red blood cells. 2000mg daily causes vomiting and gastro-intestinal upsets. 18.5mg daily can reduce blood copper levels but no physical symptoms exist. 15mg daily of zinc is considered to be a safe limit beyond which medical advice should be taken for long-term use.

INTERACTIONS AND CONTRAINDICATIONS

Zinc is linked with vitamin A to release the latter from the liver. High zinc intakes reduce levels of copper and iron, while high iron intake in turn reduces zinc levels, as do high amounts of cadmium.

iNDEX OF OTHER DIETARY SUPPLEMENTS

COENZYME Q10

Did you know?

- Coenzyme Q10 (CoQ10) occurs naturally in all human cells. CoQ10 is made in the body, but production is reduced as we get older.
- CoQ10 is also found in foods (especially meat), but cooking and processing methods tend to destroy it.
- The Japanese have been using supplemental CoQ10 for many years but it was not until 1974 that pure CoQ10 was obtained in large enough quantities for the Japanese to initiate organised trials on patients.

Therapeutic uses

- **Heart Disease** A number heart conditions have shown positive response to CoQ10. These include congestive heart failure, ischaemic heart disease, rheumatic heart disease and irregular heartbeat.
- **Periodontal (Gum) Disease** Investigations have shown that diseased gums tend to have lower levels of CoQ10 than healthy ones, and that CoQ10 supplementation can halt deterioration of the gums.
- **Weight Loss** In those who are overweight and who appear to have a CoQ10 deficiency, CoQ10 supplements may speed up weight loss. However, there is no effect in those who are not CoQ10 deficient.
- **Energy Booster** A supplement of CoQ10 does not only have benefits for people with specific health problems. Many people who simply feel tired and run down can benefit from this energy-producing nutrient. CoQ10 is also thought to act as an immune enhancer – having an antioxidant effect and directly stimulating antibody formation.

───── **SAFETY** ─────

CoQ10 is usually effective at levels of 15–60mg per day but 100mg plus has been used without any toxicity problems or side effects whatsoever.

INTERACTIONS AND CONTRAINDICATIONS

There are no known drug interactions or other contraindications for CoQ10.

---

*E*VENING PRIMROSE OIL

Did you know?

- This humble yellow flower, which is now known to possess remarkable health-giving properties was first brought to Europe from Virginia in the 1600s.
- The key to the plant's nutritional secret is the oil that is collected from its seeds.
- One of the biggest benefits of evening primrose oil is to women who suffer from premenstrual syndrome (PMS).

Benefits

- The real value of evening primrose lies in the gamma-linolenic acid (GLA) content of its oil. GLA is an important intermediary in the metabolic conversion of linoleic acid to prostaglandin E1. The normal diet is quite sufficient in the essential fatty acid linoleic acid (LA), but the first step in its conversion to prostaglandin E1 can be easily blocked. Among the known blocking agents are: viruses, carcinogens, cholesterol, saturated fatty acids, trans fatty acids, alcohol, insufficient insulin, excess dietary alpha-linolenic acid (ALA) (found in linseed and blackcurrant oils), radiation, and the ageing process.

- Traditional dietary GLA can therefore be extremely valuable since it skips these potential blockages and provides a material from which prostaglandin E1 can easily be produced.

Therapeutic uses

- **Premenstrual syndrome (PMS)** In one study, 61 per cent of PMS patients reported complete relief and 25 per cent reported partial relief when taking evening primrose oil. In another study, evening primrose oil was used with remarkable success. The symptoms of swollen abdomen and breast discomfort were eradicated in 95 per cent of the women, irritability in 80 per cent, depression in 74 per cent, swollen fingers and ankles in 79 per cent and anxiety in 53 per cent. The only two symptoms that persisted in more than half of the women were tiredness and headaches.
- **Benign breast disease** Evening primrose oil has been reported to reduce the symptoms of benign breast disease substantially. This result is attributed to the inhibition of prolactin, the same action that is effective in treating PMS.
- **Cholesterol** Evening primrose oil has been shown to lower high serum cholesterol in humans. This effect usually takes several weeks to achieve.
- **Platelet aggregation** Evening primrose oil decreases the tendency of the blood to clot.
- **Blood Pressure** Studies have shown that evening primrose oil can lower high blood pressure levels.
- **Eczema** Evening primrose oil has been used successfully in patients with atopic eczema. A study was made with adults taking either 4, 8 or 12 x 500mg capsules daily and children taking 4 or 8 x 500mg capsules daily. Results indicated that evening primrose oil brought significant clinical improvement, especially at the higher dosages.
- **Psoriasis** Psoriasis may be responsive to a combination of evening primrose oil and fish oils.
- **Multiple sclerosis (MS)** Evening primrose oil is now routinely used by multiple sclerosis sufferers with encouraging results. The unusual pattern of fatty acids that is

found in the blood cells of MS sufferers often returns to normal within a few months of taking evening primrose oil.

- **Rheumatoid arthritis** Fifty-two patients, all long-standing sufferers of arthritis and taking non-steroidal anti-inflammatory (NSAID) drugs, were given either evening primrose oil or evening primrose oil plus fish oils. 60 per cent of the patients were able to withdraw completely from NSAID treatment, and another 25 per cent were able to cut their NSAID dosage in half. Evening primrose oil with fish oils was slightly more effective than evening primrose oil alone.

- **Alcoholism** Preliminary tests in humans show evening primrose oil can make withdrawal from alcohol intake easier and can relieve post-drinking depression. Brain and liver function improve more quickly in people who have stopped drinking if they take evening primrose oil. A study of 62 alcoholics found that those taking evening primrose oil for 24 weeks had significantly faster brain function than those who were not taking it.

--------------------------------- SAFETY ---------------------------------

Evening primrose oil has very low toxicity and has been used without harm at levels of up to 5–6g daily.

INTERACTIONS AND CONTRAINDICATIONS

Evening primrose oil and fish oils can suitably be supplemented together to achieve a balance of the two families of fatty acids (omega 6 and omega 3). However, ALA and GLA/LA combinations are conflicting, as the former blocks the further conversion of the latter two. Occasionally, evening primrose oil may cause nausea, headaches or skin eruptions when first taken. This symptom quickly subsides over a period of time and can be lessened by taking the dosage with a meal.

Evening primrose oil should be avoided by epileptics as it may exacerbate a certain type of temporal lobe epilepsy.

Also, evening primrose oil is best not taken with the drugs methotrimeprazine and procarbazine, both of which depress the central nervous system. Evening primrose oil should be avoided by those taking blood-thinning drugs, such as warfarin.

*f*ISH OILS

Did you know

- The importance of omega 3 in fish oils was discovered when it was identified that Eskimos have very low blood cholesterol levels despite a diet that includes the highest animal fat content of any diet in the world.
- Sounding like something right out of science fiction, omega 3 is certainly far from fiction. It is a name given to a group of essential fatty acids that are derived primarily from oily fish, such as mackerel, salmon and herring.
- They are called 'essential' because the body can not manufacture them and they must therefore come from the diet. Fish acquire them from algae and phytoplankton.
- The omega 3 fatty acids in fish are: eicosapentaenoic acid (EPA), docosapentaenoic acid (DPA) and docosahexaenoic acid (DHA).
- The omega 3 fatty acids have been found to have the ability of reducing a group of fats called triglycerides. High levels of triglycerides impair the body's ability to break down blood clots which contribute to the risk of heart attacks.

Benefits

- A twenty-year-old study in Holland (1960–80), which involved middle-aged men without a history of coronary heart disease, demonstrated that those who consumed at least 1.1 oz of fish a day had only half the mortality rate from heart attacks as those who ate no fish.

97

- In Bristol in 1983, a study was set up to determine whether men who had already suffered a heart attack could reduce the risk of further attacks by a change in their diet. The results demonstrated that men who had increased their consumption of fatty fish had 29 per cent fewer deaths than the group that did not.
- Fish oils have been found to have significant benefits on the heart by altering the balance of blood fats in a favourable way: reducing the likelihood of blood clotting; making the heart less prone to arrhythmias (irregular heartbeats); reducing the viscosity of the blood, therefore facilitating blood flow.
- An important area of research is the link between essential fatty acids, birth weight and IQ. Babies need both omega 3 and omega 6 (found in vegetable oils) for development.

Therapeutic uses

- The use of fish oil concentrates on sufferers of rheumatoid arthritis has been shown to reduce the symptoms of swollen and tender joints, morning stiffness and pain.
- Eczema, acne and psoriasis have all been found to have improved by the increase of fish oils in the diet.

--- **SAFETY** ---

Fish oil has been used in very high amounts in clinical research without any overt toxicity symptoms. However, therapeutic levels of fish oil intake should be monitored by a medical professional, because omega 3 fatty acids can displace omega 6 fatty acids from cell membranes. There may also be a thinning of the blood and a reduction in clotting time.

INTERACTIONS AND CONTRAINDICATIONS

Fish oils and evening primrose oil can suitably be supplemented together to achieve a balance of the two families of fatty acids (omega 6 and omega 3). However, ALA and GLA/LA combinations are conflicting, as the former blocks the further conversion of the latter two.

Occasionally, fish oils may cause nausea when first taken. This symptom quickly subsides over a period of time and can be lessened by taking the dosage with a meal.

Fish oils should be avoided by those on blood-thinning drugs, such as warfarin.

$\mathcal{G}$ARLIC

Did you know?

- An Egyptian papyrus of around 1550BC includes 22 therapeutic recipes that use garlic for complaints ranging from bites to heart problems and tumours.
- The Greeks, Romans and Vikings have all left evidence that garlic was prescribed both as a preventative medicine and a cure for a variety of illnesses.
- Thousands of years use, coupled with modern scientific research, has shown garlic to be a herb with important health properties.
- Intact raw garlic cells contain alliin (an amino acid) and alliinase (an enzyme). When garlic is cut or crushed, alliin and alliinase immediately react together to produce the pungent substance allicin. Allicin kills all sorts of cells, including germs.
- Traditional Chinese herbalists prescribed garlic cloves, aged for two to three years in vinegar, to help many complaints. Today, cold-aged garlic is in principle similar to this ancient remedy.

Therapeutic uses

- Very many research papers have demonstrated the therapeutic benefits of garlic – normally at levels of around 1000mg per day. Lower doses are to be used for maintenance of general good health, rather than tackling existing ailments.
- **Cholesterol** Aged garlic can help to decrease total cholesterol while increasing HDL ('good') cholesterol.
- **Protection against free radicals and oxidation** Raw garlic is actually an oxidant rather than an antioxidant. However, the cold-ageing process reverses this and turns garlic into a strong antioxidant.
- **Anti-infection effects of garlic** Garlic's sulphur compounds are antifungal and antibacterial, which makes it effective in numerous health problems like colds and 'flu.
- Garlic has been shown to boost the activity of the body's natural killer cells and many other aspects of the immune system.
- The sulphur compounds in garlic protect against free radicals which are hazardous to health if unchecked.
- **Candida** Garlic can increase the speed of clearance of *Candida albicans* cells from the body. (Candida albicans is a yeast organism that can over-grow the digestive tract causing digestive upset, bloating, thrush, etc).
- **Respiratory problems** Garlic is suitable for use in catarrhal, respiratory or bronchial conditions.

SAFETY

Garlic has been tested extensively for toxicity, and no amount of it seems to cause side effects.

INTERACTIONS AND CONTRAINDICATIONS

There are no known drug interactions or contraindications for garlic.

g INSENG

Did you know?

- Ginseng is renowned for its alleged aphrodisiac qualities among Westerners and those from the Orient.
- In the East, however, ginseng has been used for centuries as a general medicine and has different effects for different people.
- There are two types of ginseng: *panax* which is considered to be the genuine article, and *eleutheroccus* or Siberian ginseng, which is botanically different from panax ginseng but which shares the same effects.
- Russian scientists tested ginseng on proofreaders who need good concentration powers with high accuracy and speed. Those using ginseng increased their speed by 12 per cent and decreased mistakes by an amazing 51 per cent in comparison with the readers who did not use ginseng.
- In Sweden university students undergoing exams were shown to do better when taking ginseng, while in this country nurses changing from day to night shifts found that, if taking ginseng, problems of moodiness, insomnia and decreased alertness were relieved.

Benefits

- Some definitive health benefits derived from taking ginseng: are: improved stamina, concentration, resistance to stress, disease, fatigue and protection against radiation.
- Ginseng appears to stimulate the nervous system, speeding up reflexes and increasing speed and accuracy.
- Tests have also shown an increase in learning retention.
- Ginseng, especially Siberian ginseng, differs from other stimulants, such as caffeine, in that it does not produce the side effects of jitteriness, over-stimulation or subsequent exhaustion.
- Ginseng has been shown to reverse and block the effects of alcohol and sedative drugs and also has a calming effect, and

for this reason is commonly used to alleviate stress.

Therapeutic uses

- A major study over several months involving 60,000 Soviet car workers showed that use of ginseng produced an improvement in general health.
- Japanese research scientists found that ginseng seems to strengthen the immune system.
- Ginseng has even been found to help diabetics.

--------------------------------- **SAFETY** ---------------------------------

Ginseng does not have any reported side effects.

INTERACTIONS AND CONTRAINDICATIONS

There are no known drug interactions or contraindications for ginseng.

*l*ECITHIN

Did you know?

- Lecithin is made by the liver but is also found in egg yolk and was first isolated in 1850.
- A common ingredient found in many food products, lecithin has the ability to combine oil with water-based ingredients.
- However, lecithin has earned itself a reputation as a vital factor in the prevention and treatment of heart disease, and as a positive slimming aid.
- A complex mixture of fats and essential fatty acids, lecithin itself is predominantly fat, combined with phosphorus and choline.

Benefits

- Research has shown that atherosclerosis (hardening of the arteries) can be reversed via reduction of blood cholesterol and lipids to normal levels.
- Pure soya bean lecithin, when regularly incorporated into the diet, lowers cholesterol. Lecithin and cholesterol coexist in equilibrium, with lecithin controlling cholesterol.
- As an emulsifier, lecithin breaks down fat; large particles of fat act as a landing stage where sticky platelets collect, which goes on to reduce blood circulation and eventually leads to blood clots.
- Various studies on sufferers of coronary heart disease have shown low levels of blood lecithin, with corresponding increased risk of blood clotting.
- We all know someone who can eat like a horse and stays slim while someone else just has to look at a lettuce leaf and puts on a stone! The body's metabolism is the reason behind this. Soya lecithin keeps fat from forming deposits, breaking it up into particles which can be metabolised more easily and thoroughly than large particles; lecithin prevents fat build-up.

Therapeutic uses

- **Gallstones** Lecithin is able to increase the capacity of the bile to solubilise cholesterol. At a minimum dose of 2g per day, lecithin can help to normalise the low phospholipid to cholesterol ratios found in gallstone patients.
- **Senile dementia** There have been many conflicting trials on the use of lecithin in senile dementia. However, a trial in 1985 showed that lecithin at high levels benefited a small number of patients with advanced Alzheimer's disease by improving orientation, learning and memory.
- **Multiple sclerosis (MS)** There is some evidence that the lecithin content of myelin is depleted in MS sufferers. Lecithin or choline supplements may help to slow the deterioration of the nerve coverings.

———————————————————— **SAFETY** ————————————————————

Lecithin does not have any reported side effects at levels up to
100g per day for up to four months.

INTERACTIONS AND CONTRAINDICATIONS

In Alzheimer's patients taking drugs for this condition, lecithin
may cause gastro-intestinal disturbances.

---

*R*OYAL JELLY

Did you know

- Royal jelly is produced by worker bees for consumption by
  the queen bee. There are three types of bee in a hive: the
  queen, the worker and the drone. All three types of bees
  come from the same type of egg. For the first three days after
  laying, the eggs are fed the same type of food. After that the
  future queen bees are fed a special diet – the substance
  known as royal jelly.
- An analysis of royal jelly shows that it is packed with
  nutrients. Most of the B vitamins are present (thiamin,
  riboflavin, nicotinic acid, biotin, inositol, folic acid,
  pyridoxine, cobalamin, pantothenic acid), amino acids (the
  building blocks of protein), vitamin C, the minerals calcium,
  potassium, magnesium, phosphorous, sodium, iron,
  manganese, zinc and cobalt, and fatty acids, sugars,
  hormones and nucleotides. There still remains a small
  percentage of ingredients in royal jelly that have not as yet
  been identified, and royal jelly's magic ingredient which sets
  it apart from any other nutritional supplement is one of these.
- Cliff Richard, Susan Hampshire and Sebastian Coe all take
  royal jelly and attest to its very real health-giving properties.

Benefits

- Many people find that royal jelly gives them increased stamina and high energy levels.
- Royal jelly is reported to have helped in a variety of health conditions, from acne, allergies, angina, anorexia, anxiety, and arthritis through to baldness, headaches, herpes and impotence.

————————————————— **SAFETY** —————————————————

Royal jelly does not have any reported side effects.

INTERACTIONS AND CONTRAINDICATIONS

There are no known drug interactions or contraindications for ginseng.

iNDEX OF CONDITIONS

*A*CNE VULGARIS

Vitamin A
- Vitamin A strengthens protective skin (epithelial) tissue.
- Dosage: 25,000 iu per day, for short-term use.
- Those with liver and/or blood fat problems should consult a professional before taking vitamin A supplements.

Vitamin E
- Taken with vitamin A, vitamin E can reduce acne outbreaks.
- Dosage: 400 iu with 50,000 iu of vitamin A, twice a day.

Zinc
- Zinc is known to clear acne.
- Dosage: 15–30mg per day in chelated form.

Evening primrose oil
- Evening primrose oil provides essential fatty acids (GLA) to reduce inflammation of the skin.
- Dosage: 500mg per day.

*A*IDS

Vitamin A
- Vitamin A strengthens the immune system.
- Dosage: 10,000–25,000 iu per day.

Folic acid
- Studies show low levels of folic acid in AIDS patients.
- This deficiency may lead to a weakened immune system.
- Dosage: up to 1mg per day.

Vitamin C
- Vitamin C is known to inhibit the ability of the HIV virus to duplicate itself.
- Dosage: 2000–3000mg per day.

Vitamin E

- Vitamin E is beneficial in maintaining healthy cell membranes.
- Dosage: 200–800 iu per day.

Selenium

- As an antioxidant, selenium strengthens the immune system.
- Dosage: 200mcg per day.

Zinc

- As an antioxidant, zinc strengthens the immune system.
- Studies show low levels of zinc in AIDS patients.
- Dosage: 15–30mg zinc in chelated form per day.

Evening primrose oil

- Evening primrose oil provides GLA to improve immune function.
- Dosage: 1g twice or three times per day.

ALCOHOLISM

Vitamin A

- A deficiency can cause a wide variety of problems associated with alcoholism.
- Dosage: 5000–10,000 iu per day.

B vitamins

- Alcohol abuse leads to a deficiency of B-complex vitamins.
- Dosage: 100mg B-complex preparation.
- Extra niacin (B3) – 150mg three times a day.
- Extra thiamin (B1) – 100mg per day.

Vitamin C

- Vitamin C helps detoxify and clear alcohol from the body.
- Dosage: 2000–3000mg per day.

Vitamin E

- Vitamin E is an antioxidant and protects against damage to vital organs.
- Dosage: 800 iu per day.

Zinc

- Zinc is required by the body to detoxify and digest alcohol.
- Studies show zinc reduces alcohol craving.
- Dosage: 15–30mg zinc in chelated form per day.

Selenium

- Selenium works with vitamin E to protect the liver.
- Dosage: 100–200 mcg per day.

*A*LLERGIES

Cobalamin (B12) and pantothenic acid (B5)

- These vitamins are known to help allergic conditions such as asthma and dermatitis.
- Dosage: as part of a 100mg B-complex formula.

Vitamin C with bioflavinoids

- Vitamin C is an antioxidant and is also known to inhibit the release of histamines.
- Dosage: 1000–3000mg per day.

Vitamin E

- Along with vitamins A and C, vitamin E helps to boost the immune system.
- Dosage: 200–400 iu per day.

Zinc

- As an antioxidant, zinc boosts the immune system.
- Dosage: 15–30mg of zinc in chelated form per day.

*a*NAEMIA

Folic acid
- A deficiency of folic acid causes megaloblastic anaemia, where the red blood cells produced are few in number but large in size.
- Dosage: as per your doctor's recommendation.

Thiamin and riboflavin
- A deficiency of either or both of these vitamins may cause anaemia.
- Dosage: 20–30mg thiamin per day and 20mg of riboflavin.

Pyridoxine (B6)
- Pyridoxine is important in blood cell production.
- Dosage: 100mg per day.

Cobalamin (B12)
- A deficiency of cobalamin causes pernicious anaemia, a type of megaloblastic anaemia.
- Dosage: 25–100mcg per day.

Vitamin C
- Vitamin C helps the body to absorb iron.
- Dosage: 3000mg per day.

Vitamin E
- Vitamin E is an antioxidant that makes the red blood cells less fragile.
- Dosage: 800 iu per day.

Iron
- A deficiency in iron is the one that most commonly causes anaemia.
- Dosage: usually 10mg per day or as per your doctor's recommendation.

*A*THEROSCLEROSIOS

Beta carotene

- A recent study at Harvard showed that a daily intake of beta carotene helps to reduce the risk of heart disease.
- Dosage: 15mg per day.

Pyridoxine (B6)

- Without pyridoxine the build-up of an amino acid (homocysteine) in the artery walls encourages cholesterol deposits.
- Dosage: 40–50mg per day with 100mg dose B-complex.

Vitamin C

- Dr Linus Pauling's recent work has been focused on the role of vitamin C in preventing formation of cholesterol plaque in the arteries.
- Dosage: 1000mg per day.

Vitamin E

- Recent research has shown that a daily intake of vitamin E can help to reduce the risk of heart disease.
- Dosage: 200–800 iu per day.

Fish oils

- These have been found to lower LDL cholesterol and promote HDL cholesterol.
- Dosage: 1–2g per day.

Garlic

- Recent research has found that garlic beneficially affects the three most important factors for heart health – high blood pressure, high cholesterol levels and high platelet stickiness.
- Dosage: 1000mg aged garlic extract per day.

*A*RTHRITIS

Niacin (B3)

- Niacin is helpful in reducing pain and increasing the mobility of joints.
- It increases the blood flow by dilating small arteries.
- Dosage: 250mg twice a day with 100mg vitamin B-complex.

Vitamin C

- Vitamin C is a powerful antioxidant that scavenges free radicals.
- It is required for the formation of collagen – the main protein component of cartilage and bone.
- Vitamin C helps to build and repair smooth cartilage surfaces and maintain ligaments and tendons.
- Dosage: 1000–3000mg per day in divided doses.

Vitamin E

- As an antioxidant, vitamin E protects from free radical damage.
- Vitamin E helps joint mobility, particularly in osteoarthritis.
- Dosage: 400–600 iu per day.

Selenium

- As an antioxidant this mineral helps the body to make glutathione – a free radical scavenger which prevents oxidation and hence damage to joint linings.
- Dosage: 100–200 mcg per day.

Evening primrose oil and fish oils

- These supplements have been found to control inflammation of the joints.
- They are needed by the body to make prostaglandins – anti-inflammatory substances.
- Dosage: 2–3g evening primrose oil with 1–2g fish oil.

*A*STHMA

Beta carotene

- Beta carotene helps boost the immune system, so it is important for asthma caused by allergies.
- Dosage: 15mg per day.

Pyridoxine (B6)

- Asthmatics are known to have low levels of vitamin B6, particularly those on certain drugs such as theophylline.
- Dosage: 50mg per day.

Vitamin C

- As an antioxidant, vitamin C aids the immune system and is also a natural antihistamine.
- It is necessary for antibody response.
- Dosage: 1000–2000mg per day.

Vitamin E

- Vitamin E neutralises free radicals and works with other nutrients in boosting the immune system.
- 200–800 iu per day.

Selenium

- As an antioxidant this mineral helps the body to make glutathione – a free radical scavenger which prevents oxidation and hence damage to mucous membranes.
- Dosage: 200 mcg per day.

Evening primrose oil

- The gamma-linolenic acid in evening primrose oil helps to produce hormone-like anti-inflammatory substances called prostaglandins which control the exaggerated immune response in asthma.
- Dosage: 1000mg of evening primrose oil three times a day.

*b*URNS

Vitamin C
- Vitamin C is required for the formation of collagen – the main protein component of fibrous and scar tissue needed to heal burns.
- The stress of injury creates a higher demand for vitamin C.
- Dosage: 1000–3000mg per day in divided doses.

Vitamin E
- Vitamin E helps healing and is needed to prevent scarring.
- Dosage: 200–400 iu per day; may also be applied directly to the skin as oil.

Zinc
- Zinc is needed for faster healing of the skin.
- Dosage: 15–30mg per day.

*b*URSITIS

Cobalamin (B12)
- Vitamin B12 is known to reduce inflammation and pain.
- Dosage: by injection or 'under the tongue' under your doctor's supervision, with 100mg dose B-complex.

Vitamin C
- Vitamin C is used as a preventative treatment for inflammation and for boosting the immune system.
- Dosage: 1000mg per day.

Vitamin E
- As an antioxidant, vitamin E helps reduce inflammation of the bursa.
- Dosage: 400–800 iu per day.

Evening primrose oil and fish oils
- These oils have been found to control inflammation of the joints.
- They are needed by the body to make prostaglandins – anti-inflammatory substances.
- Dosage: 2–3g evening primrose oil with 1–2g fish oil per day.

CHRONIC FATIGUE SYNDROME

Vitamin B-complex
- Vitamin B-complex is required for increased energy levels.
- Dosage: 100mg three times per day.

Vitamin C
- Vitamin C has a powerful antiviral effect.
- Dosage: 1000mg per day.

Magnesium
- A magnesium deficiency causes weakness and fatigue.
- Dosage: 450mg per day.

Coenzyme Q10
- CoQ10 is known to help relieve symptoms of chronic fatigue.
- Dosage: 30mg two to three times per day.

COLD SORES

Vitamin C
- As an antioxidant, vitamin C helps to reduce the frequency of cold sore attacks and can abort outbreaks if taken early.
- Dosage: 1000mg per day.

Vitamin E
- Vitamin E enhances the healing process.
- Dosage: squeeze open a 200 iu capsule and apply to blistered areas three times a day.

Zinc

- Taken in combination with vitamin C, zinc can be beneficial in preventing recurrence of cold sore attacks.
- Dosage: 15–30mg, in chelated form, per day.

COMMON COLD

Vitamin A

- These vitamins help heal the mucous membranes as well as boosting the immune system.
- Dosage: 10,000–25,000 iu (short term) per day.

Vitamin C

- Dr Linus Pauling's work has promoted the role of vitamin C in preventing the common cold.
- Dosage: 3000mg per day.

Zinc

- Zinc can be beneficial in preventing recurrence of the cold.
- Dosage: 15mg, in chelated form, per day.

Garlic

- Garlic enhances the immune function – it is also a natural antibiotic.
- Dosage: 1000mg aged garlic extract per day.

CROHN'S DISEASE

Folic acid

- A deficiency in folic acid is common in sufferers of this disease because of poor absorption due to inflamed intestinal tissues.
- Dosage: 400–1000mcg and 100mg B-complex per day.

Vitamin C

- The need for vitamin C increases when the body is under attack and inflamed.
- Dosage: 1000mg per day.

Iron

- Loss of blood may deplete iron stores.
- Dosage: ensure adequate supply of iron-rich foods.

Magnesium

- A magnesium deficiency can be caused by poor absorption and loss during diarrhoea.
- Dosage: 200–400mg magnesium with 400–800mg calcium per day.

*d*EPRESSION

Biotin

- A deficiency of biotin is known to cause depression.
- Dosage: 300 mcg per day for 4–6 weeks.

Folic acid and pyridoxine (B6)

- A deficiency of folic acid and/or pyridoxine can contribute to changes of moods as these B vitamins are required to maintain optimum levels of the mood-elevating chemical serotonin.
- Dosage: 1g folic acid and 100mg vitamin B6 with 100mg B-complex per day.

Cynacobalamin (B12)

- More often than not, people suffering from depression are deficient in cobalamin.
- Dosage: 500 mcg with 100mg vitamin B-complex per day.

Vitamin C

- A mild deficiency of vitamin C is enough to cause chronic depression and fatigue.
- Dosage: 1000mg per day.

*d*ERMATITIS

Vitamin A and beta carotene
- Dry scaling of skin is improved with both vitamin A and beta carotene.
- Dosage: 15mg of beta carotene per day.

Vitamin B-complex
- Vitamin B-complex is required for healthy skin and proper circulation.
- Dosage: 100mg per day.

Zinc
- Zinc helps to clear rashes in some sufferers.
- Dosage: 15–30mg in chelated form three times per day.

Evening primrose oil and fish oils
- Both have been found to reduce inflammation thus inhibiting skin irritations, itching and scaling.
- Dosage: 2–3g evening primrose oil with 1g fish oil per day.

*d*IABETES MELLITUS

Vitamin B-complex
- Vitamin B-complex is important in preventing nerve damage in diabetics.
- Dosage: 100mg B-complex per day.

Chromium
- Chromium helps improve sugar metabolism, promote blood sugar control and increase energy.
- Dosage: 200mcg, in chelated form, or 10gm brewer's yeast per day.

Zinc
- A zinc deficiency impairs blood sugar control.
- Dosage: 15–30mg in chelated form three times per day.

*e*PILEPSY

Pyridoxine (B6)
- This deficiency is known to cause seizures.
- Dosage: 40–50mg per day with 100mg B-complex.

Vitamin E
- Anticonvulsant drugs cause a depletion of vitamin E.
- Dosage: 200–400 iu per day.

Magnesium
- A deficiency of magnesium increases the risk of seizures.
- Dosage: 200–400mg per day.

*f*ATIGUE

B vitamins
- B vitamins are needed for physical or emotional stress and to help energy production.
- Dosage: 100mg B-complex preparation.

Vitamin C
- Vitamin C helps concentration and relieves fatigue.
- Dosage: 500 to 1000mg per day.

Iron
- A deficiency of iron may contribute to fatigue.
- Dosage: supplement under medical supervision.

*h*AY FEVER

Beta carotene
- Beta carotene helps boost the immune system, so it is important for hay fever caused by allergies.
- Dosage: 15mg per day.

Cobalamin (B12)

- Cobalamin is known to provide relief for wheezing and is effective in increasing tolerance to allergens.
- Dosage: By injections or taken 'under the tongue' under your doctor's supervision.

Vitamin C

- As an antioxidant it aids the immune system and is also a natural antihistamine.
- Vitamin C is necessary for antibody response.
- Dosage: 1000–2000mg per day.

Vitamin E

- Vitamin E neutralises free radicals and works with other nutrients in boosting the immune system.
- Dosage: 200–800 iu per day.

Selenium

- As an antioxidant this mineral helps the body to make glutathione – a free radical scavenger which prevents oxidation and hence damage to mucous membranes.
- Dosage: 200 mcg per day.

*h*EADACHES AND MIGRAINES

Niacin (B3)

- Niacin is known for its vasodilatory effects and is used in the treatment of migraines.
- Dosage: 100mg per day.

Magnesium

- Magnesium is beneficial in relaxing muscles.
- Dosage: 500mg per day.

Fish oil

- Increasing consumption of fish oil has been known to help migraine victims.
- Dosage: 2g fish oil per day.

hEAVY PERIODS

Vitamin A or beta carotene
- Women with excessive bleeding may have a marginal deficiency of vitamin A.
- Dosage: 25,000 iu vitamin A or 15mg beta carotene (for not more than two weeks).

Vitamin C with bioflavinoids
- This vitamin helps reduce heavy blood flow.
- Dosage: 500mg twice a day.

Iron
- Iron reduces heavy bleeding.
- Dosage: 30mg per day in chelated form.

hEPATITIS

B-complex vitamins
- B vitamins are needed to enhance normal liver function.
- Dosage: 100mg B-complex .

Vitamin C
- Vitamin C helps to boost the immune function, particularly when under attack from virus.
- Dosage: 2000mg per day.

Vitamin E
- Sufferers of hepatitis are found to be deficient in vitamin E, thus leading to weakening of the immune system.
- Dosage: 800 iu per day.

Selenium
- As an antioxidant, selenium helps the immune system in countering viral attack.
- Dosage: 100–200 mcg per day.

*h*IGH BLOOD PRESSURE

Beta carotene
- A deficiency of beta carotene can contribute to high blood pressure.
- Dosage: 15mg per day.

Vitamin D
- Vitamin D is known to assist in the absorption of calcium and hence help reduce blood pressure.
- Plenty of sunshine will allow the body to make enough of this vitamin.

Magnesium and calcium
- Low calcium levels increase the risk of high blood pressure.
- Magnesium can help reduce blood pressure as it has the ability to relax and, therefore, widen blood vessels.
- Dosage: 200–400mg magnesium with 400–800mg calcium per day.

Garlic
- Garlic is known to be beneficial in lowering blood pressure.
- Dosage: 1000mg of aged garlic extract per day.

*i*MPOTENCE

Vitamin C
- Makes the sperm more motile. Protects against free radical damage.
- Dosage: 1000mg per day.

Zinc
- A deficiency in zinc is known to be a contributing cause of impotency.
- Dosage: 15–30mg per day.

*i*NFERTILITY – MALE

Cynacobalamin (B12)

- Cynacobalamin helps increase a low sperm count and increases sperm motility.
- Dosage: 100mg B-complex. Separate 'under the tongue' intake under supervision of a health professional.

Vitamin C

- As an antioxidant, vitamin C protects the sperm from oxidation, especially in the female reproductive tract. It is also known to boost sperm count.
- Dosage: 1000mg per day.

Vitamin E

- Vitamin E is required for balanced hormone production.
- Dosage: 200–400 iu per day.

Selenium

- There is speculation that selenium plays a part in increasing the chances of conception since it helps the body in producing glutathione peroxide, a natural antioxidant that can protect the sperm in its passage through the female reproductive tract.
- Dosage: 200 mcg per day.

Zinc

- Low levels of zinc are known to reduce production of the male hormone, testosterone.
- Dosage: 15–30mg per day.

*i*NFERTILITY – FEMALE

Folic acid
- A deficiency in folic acid is attributed to difficulty in conceiving.
- Dosage: 1–2mg folic acid with 50mg B-complex vitamin B12.

Pyridoxine (B6)
- This vitamin helps increase female reproductive hormone, progesterone.
- Dosage: 50–100mg per day.

*i*NFLAMMATION

Vitamin C
- Vitamin C minimises inflammation caused by injury or infection.
- Dosage: 1000mg per day.

Vitamin E
- As an antioxidant, vitamin E helps to reduce inflammation.
- Dosage: 400 iu per day.

Copper and zinc
- Both are required for the production of the body's own antioxidant called superoxide dismutase (SOD).
- Dosage: 15mg zinc and 1–2mg copper in chelated form per day.

Selenium
- As an antioxidant this mineral helps the body to make glutathione, a free radical scavenger which helps curb inflammation.
- Dosage: 200 mcg per day

Evening primrose oil & fish oils

- These supplements are important in controlling inflammatory response.
- Dosage: 2–3g evening primrose oil with 1–2g fish oil per day.

*k*IDNEY STONES

Pyridoxine (B6)

- Pyridoxine is necessary for breaking down oxalic acid.
- Dosage: 50–100mg per day.

Magnesium

- Low levels of magnesium are also known to contribute to the formation of kidney stones.
- Dosage: 400mg per day.

*m*ENOPAUSE

Pyridoxine (B6)

- Pyridoxine helps to reduce water retention.
- Dosage: 50–100mg per day.

Vitamin C with bioflavinoids

- This vitamin helps relieve hot flushes.
- Dosage: 1000mg per day.

Vitamin E

- Vitamin E helps to reduce fatigue and, in some cases, menopausal headaches.
- Dosage: 400 iu per day.

Evening primrose oil

- This supplement is important in keeping a healthy hormone balance.
- Dosage: 1g evening primrose oil three times a day.

*M*USCLE WEAKNESS

Riboflavin (B2)
- Riboflavin helps to relieve the weakness caused by reduced energy production.
- Dosage: 50–100mg per day with 100mg B-complex formula.

Vitamin C
- Vitamin C helps to release energy from cells, the lack of which causes weakness of the muscles.
- Dosage: 1000–2000mg per day.

Magnesium
- A deficiency of magnesium is known to cause muscle weakness.
- Dosage: 250mg per day.

*N*AIL PROBLEMS

Calcium and magnesium
- A deficiency of calcium is a common cause of brittle nails. For the most effective results, supplement calcium with magnesium.
- Dosage: 100mg calcium with 500mg magnesium.

Vitamin C
- Vitamin C is useful in cases of inflammation of the tissue surrounding the nail.
- Dosage: 1000–2000mg per day.

Iron
- A deficiency of iron can cause brittle nails.
- Dosage: 10mg iron in chelated form per day.

Zinc
- A deficiency of zinc can be a cause of brittle nails.
- Dosage: 15–30mg zinc in chelated form, daily.

Evening primrose oil and fish oils
- These oils help to reduce the brittleness of nails.
- Dosage: 2–3g evening primrose oil with 1–2g fish oil per day.

*O*EDEMA

Pyridoxine (B6)
- Pyridoxine helps to reduce water retention.
- Dosage: 100mg per day with 100mg B-complex.

Vitamin C with bioflavinoids
- This vitamin helps prevent capillary weakness due to which fluid leaks out from the bloodstream into the body tissue, which in turn causes swelling of hands and feet.
- Dosage: 2000mg per day.

Vitamin E
- Vitamin E is useful in blocking increased swelling especially when linked to allergies.
- Dosage: 100–400 iu per day.

*O*STEOPOROSIS

Folic acid
- Folic acid is required for a strong bone framework.
- Dosage: 800mcg per day with 100mg B-complex.

Pyridoxine (B6)
- Vitamin D is required for building fibrous bone framework.
- Dosage: 50mg per day with 100mg B-complex.

Vitamin D
- Vitamin D is needed for calcium absorption from the intestine.
- Dosage: 2mg (800 iu) per day.

Magnesium and calcium

- A deficiency of calcium is known to contribute towards osteoporosis. Magnesium helps to activate the chemical reaction necessary for bone formation.
- Dosage: 400mg magnesium with 400–800mg calcium per day.

$\mathcal{P}$ARKINSON'S DISEASE

Niacin (B3)

- Niacin improves brain circulation.
- Dosage: 100mg per day with 100mg B-complex.

Pyridoxine (B6)

- Pyridoxine is required for the conversion of dopamine – the deficiency of which causes the condition.
- Dosage: under doctor's supervision.

Vitamin C

- Vitamin C helps to mitigate the side effects of medications for Parkinson's disease, and also improves circulation in the brain.
- Dosage: 2000mg per day.

Vitamin E

- Vitamin E prevents oxidative damage to part of the brain and hence reduces the likelihood of developing this disease.
- Dosage: 400 iu per day.

Evening primrose oil and fish oils

- The gamma-linolenic acid in evening primrose oil helps to produce hormone-like anti-inflammatory substances called prostaglandin which control the hand tremors in sufferers.
- Dosage: 2–3g evening primrose oil with 1–2g fish oil per day.

*P*REGNANCY

Folic acid
- Folic acid is shown to reduce the occurence of birth defects related to the spinal canal.
- Dosage: 400mcg per day.

Vitamin E
- Vitamin E is beneficial in reducing the risk of pre-eclampsia (fluid retention and high blood pressure).
- Dosage: 100 to 200 iu per day.

Zinc
- The level of zinc often declines during pregnancy.
- A deficiency of zinc can lead to a higher risk of miscarriage, premature delivery and low birth weight babies.
- Dosage: 15mg zinc in chelated form per day.

Evening primrose oil
- This supplement is particularly helpful to those who have problems of fluid retention during pregnancy.
- Dosage: 2g per day.

*P*REMENSTRUAL SYNDROME (PMS)

Pyridoxine (B6)
- Pyridoxine is known to reduce the emotional symptoms of PMS.
- Dosage: 40–50mg per day with 100mg B-complex.

Magnesium
- A deficiency of magnesium can contribute to emotional symptoms as it can cause the levels of brain chemicals to fall.
- Dosage: 200–400mg per day.

Evening primrose oil

- The gamma-linolenic acid in evening primrose oil helps to produce hormone-like substances called prostaglandins, which are widely believed to play an important role in relieving fluid retention, headaches and mood swings, among other symptoms of PMS.
- Dosage: 1g evening primrose oil three times a day.

*P*SORIASIS

Vitamin A

- Sufferers of psoriasis are found to have a marginal deficiency of vitamin A.
- Dosage: 10,000–25,000 iu (short term) per day.

Vitamin D

- Vitamin D can help to alleviate the rash that accompanies this condition.
- Sunshine or ultraviolet light can be sufficient for the body to produce vitamin D.

Selenium

- Selenium is required to produce glutathione peroxide – the body's own antioxidant which can control inflammation.
- Dosage: 200mcg per day .

Evening primrose oil

- Evening primrose oil provides essential fatty acids (GLA) to improve inflammation.
- Dosage: 1000mg three times per day.

Fish oil

- Provides essential fatty acids to improve inflammation.
- Dosage: 1–2g per day.

*S*TRESS

B-complex

- B-complex vitamins are important in alleviating symptoms of stress.
- Dosage: 100mg of B-complex twice a day.

Vitamin C

- An extra quantity of vitamin C is required for those under stress.
- Dosage: 500–1000mg per day.

*U*RTICARIA (HIVES)

Niacin (B3)

- Niacin helps to control the release of histamines.
- Dosage: 250mg per day with 100mg B-complex.

Vitamin C with bioflavinoids

- This vitamin reduces the severity of allergic swelling by decreasing the leakiness of capillaries.
- Dosage: 500mg twice a day.

Magnesium

- A deficiency of magnesium is known to increase urticaria.
- Dosage: 200–400mg magnesium with 400–800mg calcium per day.

*W*EAKENED IMMUNE SYSTEM

Beta carotene
- Beta carotene strengthens the immune system deficiency which impairs the body's defence mechanism.
- Dosage: 15mg per day.

Pyridoxine (B6)
- Pyridoxine is needed to build new immune fighters.
- Dosage: 20–50mg per day with 100mg B-complex.

Cobalamin (B12)
- A cobalamin deficiency weakens the response of immune defenders.
- Dosage: 'under the tongue' intake of cobalamin under supervision of a health professional.

Vitamin C
- Vitamin C is widely recognised as being effective in boosting the immune function and helping to resist invasion by bacteria, viruses, etc.
- Dosage: 1000mg per day.

Vitamin E
- A deficiency of vitamin E impairs the immune function and acts as a free radical scavenger along with vitamins A and C.
- Dosage: 200–400 iu per day.

Selenium
- As an antioxidant, selenium strengthens the immune system. A deficiency hinders antibody production.
- Dosage: 200mcg per day.

Zinc
- As an antioxidant, zinc improves the response from the immune system.
- Dosage: 15–30mg zinc in chelated form per day.

$\mathcal{G}$ LOSSARY

Absorption The process of incorporating food nutrients into the body through the intestine.

Active transport An energy requiring absorption process used to facilitate the entry of important biomolecules such as glucose and amino acids.

Adipose tissue Fats are stored in these body tissues.

Amino acid A characteristic group of 22 compounds sharing the ability to link together in chain formations to form proteins.

Amino acid, essential An amino acid which the body cannot make by itself and must be supplied in the diet. There are eight: methionine, threonine, tryptophan, isoleucine, leucine, lysine, valine and phenylalanine.

Anabolic The process where living cells convert simpler substances into more complex compounds.

Anaemia A condition of the blood characterised by too few red blood cells.

Anorexia A psychologically derived inability or refusal to eat.

Antioxidant A substance capable of protecting cells and body tissue from oxidation.

Artery A vessel carrying oxygenated blood away from the heart.

Atherosclerosis The progressive clogging of the arteries by fats and minerals thus constricting the flow of blood.

Arthritis Inflammation of the joints.

Bile A natural fat-emulsifying compound produced by the liver to assist dietary fat absorption.

Bile acid A component of bile derived from cholesterol.

Bioflavonoids Water-soluble companions of vitamin C.

Bulimia The wilful regurgitation of meals to control weight. Often accompanied with anorexia.

Calorie A unit of heat energy used to describe the energy content of foods.

Cancer The malignant growth of cells uncontrolled by normal regulation mechanisms which can be spread throughout the body killing the host.

Carbohydrate An energy containing molecule consisting of carbon, hydrogen, and oxygen. Humans use glucose and starch composed of many glucose molecules as a primary carbohydrate source.

Carotene A yellow pigment that may be converted into vitamin A in the body.

Catabolic The process of tearing down tissues to supply energy or molecules for other structures, as in post-surgical tissue repair.

Catalyst A chemical or molecule which acts to facilitate a chemical reaction. Enzymes are protein molecules that act as catalysts for almost every reaction in the body. Vitamins are catalysts and act as co-factors for many energy-releasing reactions in the body.

Cholesterol A waxy, fatty substance which is an essential component of every living cell wall. Transported around the body in blood.

Clotting The process of blood cell aggregation and solidification which is necessary to prevent blood loss in trauma, but which

becomes a hazard for narrowed blood vessels in the legs, brain and heart.

Coenzymes Substances that work with body enzymes.

Collagen An abundant structural protein found throughout the body, including tendons, ligaments, skin, etc.

Density, nutrient The ratio of a food's nutrient content versus the food energy (calories) it contains.

Diabetes A disease of carbohydrate metabolism where blood glucose cannot be efficiently absorbed and tissues are deprived of the energy. Additionally, the too high level of glucose becomes a health threat over time because of chemical changes in various tissues.

Diet The totality of what a person eats. Also, a recommended set of instructions by which a person should make food choices.

Diffusion, passive The process of a molecule passing from one side of a barrier (cell wall) to the other by virtue of a greater concentration on one side than the other.

Diverticulosis The inflammation of intestinal

outpouchings or 'diverticula' most often caused by straining at stool from a low fibre diet.

Eating Disorder A psychological state or condition which affects a person's ability to make proper food choices.

Enzyme A protein molecule made of a specific sequence of amino acids and possessing a unique structure for the purpose of facilitating biochemical reactions.

EPA (eicosapentaenoic acid) An essential fatty acid derived from fish oils.

Epithelial cell A specific cell type found in the outermost layer of the mucous membranes lining the digestive, respiratory and urinary tracts.

Essential amino acid Any of the 8 amino acids which the human body cannot make for itself from other molecules. These include: tryptophan, phenylalanine, leucine, isoleucine, threonine, methionine, lysine and valine.

Fat The lipid form of energy storage, consisting of triglycerides, which consist of a glycerol molecule attached to three fatty acid molecules.

Fat, saturated Triglyceride where all three fatty acids contain no unsaturated double bonds.

Fat, monounsaturated Triglyceride where the fatty acid molecules have two hydrogen atoms missing. This molecule is therefore said to contain one double bond.

Fat, polyunsaturated Triglyceride composed of fatty acids which has two or more hydrogen atoms missing. The molecule is therefore said to contain two, three, or four, double bonds.

Fatty acid A molecule comprised of a carbon chain and hydrogen atoms attached to the carbon atoms. The number of carbon atoms in the chain will determine the physical characteristics of the fatty acid and the triglyceride it is attached to.

Fibre The non-digestible portion of plant foods which serves to retain water and provide for a more easily moved food mass through the intestinal tract.

Free radical A highly chemical reactive molecule generated from the decomposition of unsaturated fatty acids.

HDL High density lipoprotein or the type of cholesterol which helps transport fats to the liver for processing and serves to keep arteries clear.

Heart disease The general premature failure of the heart and circulatory system from overconsumption of food, especially fats and the underconsumption of antioxidant nutrients from fruits and vegetables.

Heme iron Highly absorbable animal-source iron bound to a Heme molecule in haemoglobin or myoglobin.

Haemoglobin The iron-containing oxygen-carrying molecule in red blood cells.

High density lipoprotein *See* HDL.

Histamine A common chemical messenger released during cell damage (in allergies), which stimulates stomach acid secretion.

Hypervitaminosis The overconsumption of any one vitamin resulting in actual or potential harm for the individual.

Hypovitaminosis The underconsumption of any one vitamin resulting in actual or potential harm for the individual.

Immune suppression Any force or factor which diminishes the effectiveness of the immune system. The immune system is easily damaged by oxidized fats.

Immune system The collective grouping of cells, tissues and glands which police the body for foreign invaders such as food protein, bacteria, viruses and fungi.

International unit (iu) A measure of vitamin A (or E) activity that is internationally understood in the scientific community. These measurements were once done by biological assay, but today are done by chemical analysis. Ten iu of plant form Vitamin A is equal to 1 Retinol Equivalent, and 3.33 iu from animal form Vitamin A equals 1 Retinol Equivalent. The average of 5 iu from combined plant and animal Vitamin A sources equals 1 Retinol Equivalent is also used.

Intestine, small The section of the intestinal tract directly after the stomach and directly before the large intestine or colon where digestion and absorption occurs.

Intestine, large The section of the intestinal tract directly after the small intestine and before the anus, also known as the colon, where electrolytes and water are absorbed.

KCAL (kilocalorie) A unit used to measure the energy value of food. 1kcal=1000 calories.

Lactation The production of mother's milk beginning immediately after birth for the nourishment of the newborn.

LDL Stands for low density lipoprotein, the fraction of cholesterol which deposits fats on to the artery walls.

Lifestyle Any specific or group of behaviours that may affect an individual's health.

Lifestyle factor A specific behaviour or circumstance which may affect an individual's health.

Lipid Descriptive of fat-like qualities to a substance or molecule.

Lipoprotein A complex of lipids and proteins which transport lipids in the blood.

Low density Lipoprotein *See* LDL.

Macronutrient A nutrient, generally proteins, carbohydrates and fats, required daily in substantial quantities for the promotion of good health.

Malabsorption An irreglar inability to absorb a nutrient or class of nutrients often leading to further problems.

Megadose A supplemental amount of a nutrient well in excess of physiological needs.

Megaloblastic anaemia A disease of the blood characterised by enlarged immature red blood cells in the bone marrow.

Metabolism The sum of the processes in the building up and breaking down of the substances in the body.

Micronutrient A nutrient, generally vitamins and minerals, required daily in small amounts for the promotion of good health.

Mineral A chemical element nutrient not of animal or vegetable origin.

Monounsaturated fat *See* Fat, Monounsaturated.

Myoglobin The oxygen-carrying molecule in the muscle tissue.

Natural Of natural origin, commonly used to describe nutrients.

Neurotransmitter A class of chemicals used by the nervous system to communicate information within and externally to the central nervous system.

Nutrient A chemical or class of chemicals which the human body cannot create for itself and must therefore obtain from the diet.

Nutrient density *See* Density, Nutrient.

Oxidative stress The increased demand on the body's antioxidant systems caused by the increased metabolism of exercise, or by free radical damage.

Pernicious anaemia A disease of the blood caused by the absence of or the inability to absorb cobalamin (vitamin B12).

Polyunsaturated fat *See* Fat, Polyunsaturated.

Protein Any of numerous molecules in the body composed of variable sequences of 22 amino acids. Proteins are found as structures (collagen, keratin): information-carrying molecules (hormones, peptides) and immune system molecules (globulins).

Provitamin The precursor form of a nutrient which is later activated into the final form. Beta carotene is the provitamin form of vitamin A and is found in plants.

Retinol equivalent A measure of vitamin A activity: the amount of retinol that a vitamin A compound will yield after conversion. 1 RE=3.33 iu from animal foods and 1 RE=10 iu from plant foods (*see* International Unit).

Saturated fat *See* Fat, Saturated.

Supplement A nutrient taken in addition to food sources usually in a liquid, pill or powder form.

Supplementation The regular use of supplements.

Synthetic Man-made or assembled from smaller components usually in large-scale chemical manufacturing plants.

Synthesise The process of assembly from smaller components into larger molecules.

Tissue A group of cells formed together for a specialised function.

Toxic Representing immediate or long-term harmful potential to the human organism.

Triglyceride An assembly of a carbon glycerol backbone to which is attached three fatty acids of various composition.

Vegan A vegetarian who consumes only plant foods, and no dairy, eggs, fish or flesh.

Vegetarian A loose description of one who limits or omits animal foods from their diet:

-lacto-ovo- a vegetarian who consumes only milk and eggs in addition to plant foods; *-ovo-* a vegetarian who consumes only eggs and plant foods, omitting flesh, fish and dairy; *-pesco-* a vegetarian who consumes fish and plant foods, omitting flesh, eggs and dairy; *-vegan-* a vegetarian consuming only plant foods;

Vitamin Any of a group of organic chemicals necessary for the normal metabolic functioning of the body.

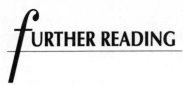URTHER READING

Vitamin Guide by Hasnain Walji (Element Books) 1992

E for Additives by Maurice Hanssen (Thorsons) 1988

The VItamin Bible by Dr Earl Mindell (Arlington Books) 1991

Vitamins and Your Health by Ann Gildroy (Unwin) 1982

Vitamin Vitality by Patrick Holford (Collins) 1985

Complete Nutrition by Dr Michael Sharon (Prion) 1989

Beta Carotene by Caroline Wheater (Thorsons) 1991

The Premenstrual Syndrome by Dr Caroline Shreeve (Thorsons) 1983

The University Of California San Diego Nutrition Book by Paul Saltman, Joel Gurin and Ira Mothner (Little, Brown and Company) 1987

$\mathcal{U}$SEFUL ADDRESSES

The British Society for Nutritional Medicine, 4 Museum Street, York, YO1 2ES, maintains a register of qualified medical professionals as well as associate members who are qualified members of the related professions.

The British Naturopathic and Osteopathic Association, 6 Netherall Gardens, London, NW3 5RR, maintains a register of qualified practitioners who have followed a four-year course at the British College of Naturopathy and Osteopathy.

The Nutrition Association, 36 Wycombe Road, Marlow, Buckinghamshire, SL7 3HX; The Nutrition Consultants Association, c/o The Institute of Optimum Nutrition, 5 Jerdan Street, London, SW6 1BE; The Society for the Promotion of Nutritional Therapy, First Floor, The Enterprise Centre, Station Parade, Eastbourne, BN1 1BE; maintain a register of practitioners of nutrition and diet therapy.

$\mathcal{A}$UTHOR PROFILE

Hasnain Walji is a researcher, writer and freelance journalist specialising in holistic health, nutrition and complementary therapies. A contributor to several journals on environmental and Third World consumer issues, he was the founder and editor of *The Vitamin Connection – An International Journal of Nutrition, Health and Fitness*, published in the UK, Canada and Australia, focusing on the link between health and diet. He also launched Healthy Eating, a consumer magazine focusing on the concept of optimum nutrition and has written a script for a six-part television series, *The World of Vitamins*, shortly to be produced by a Danish Television company. He is the author of *The Vitamin Guide – Essential Nutrients for Healthy Living*, published by Element Books as part of their *Health Essentials* series.

Hasnain has also written six books as part of a new series exploring common ailments from complementary and orthodox points of view under the Headway *Healthwise* series published by Hodder & Stoughton, and endorsed by the Natural Medicines Society of the United Kingdom. The titles are: *Asthma and Hay Fever; Skin Conditions; Alcohol, Smoking, Tranquillisers; Headaches and Migraine; Arthritis and Rheumatism; Heart Health*.

He is Vice President – Research & Development – of Software Development Innovations Inc. (Dallas, Texas), the publishers and developers of NutriPlus™ and has been responsible for co-ordinating research, design and development of this nutrition database and diet analysis program from the outset.